2/06

3
5/6/204

D1112213

37334

UNDERSTANDING
GENETICS

• • • • • • • • • • •

Myths about Inheritance and Birth Defects

Myth: Blue eye color is recessive to brown eye color. Blue-eyed parents cannot have a brown-eyed child.

Fact: Eye color is not controlled by just one gene. Inheritance of eye color is as complex as inheritance of skin color or height.

Myth: Birth defects are caused by things that the mother sees or hears.

Fact: There are many superstitions about what causes birth defects. Increasingly, the true cause can be identified. Birth defects are neither caused nor prevented by supernatural, astrologic phenomenon or by maternal experiences.

Myth: The fetus is protected by the placenta from anything that happens to the mother.

Fact: The placenta is not a strong barrier. The fetus is exposed to all the same things to which the mother is exposed. Maternal alcohol intake causes mental retardation. Maternal smoking causes growth retardation. Some fetal problems can be treated by giving medication to the mother.

Myth: If the problem is not present at birth, it isn't genetic.

Fact: Genetic diseases can be diagnosed at any age.

Myth: All genetic disease happens in childhood.

Fact: While genetic diseases and birth defects are most significant in childhood, genetic problems can manifest at any age.

Myth: All problems present at birth are genetic.

Fact: Infections, chemicals, and other things can cause problems that are present at birth.

Myth: It is only genetic if someone else in the family has it, too.

Fact: Conditions can be hidden, or very mild, or cause problems that are not talked about, and they are all equally genetic.

Myth: All persons with genetic disease or birth defect are mentally retarded or disabled.

Fact: There is a wide spectrum. Some conditions can be managed with diet, medications, or surgery. Some conditions cause no real problem at all.

Myth: Using infertility treatments lowers my risk of having a child with a birth defect.

Fact: A child conceived with infertility treatments is at the same general risk as a child conceived naturally. Some assisted reproductive techniques may contribute to passing on genetic disease.

Myth: Now that the human genome is sequenced, we know everything.

Fact: Sequencing the genome is the end of the beginning, rather than the beginning of the end.

UNDERSTANDING
GENETICS

• • • • • • • • • • •

A Primer for Couples and Families

Angela Scheuerle, M.D.

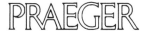

Westport, Connecticut
London

Library of Congress Cataloging-in-Publication Data

Scheuerle, Angela.
  Understanding genetics : a primer for couples and families / Angela Scheuerle.
    p. cm.
  Includes bibliographical references and index.
  ISBN 0–275–98189–4 (alk. paper)
  1. Medical genetics—Popular works.   I. Title.
    RB155.S283   2005
    616′.042—dc22   2004028072

British Library Cataloguing in Publication Data is available.

Library of Congress Catalog Card Number: 2004028072
ISBN: 0–275–98189–4

First published in 2005

Praeger Publishers, 88 Post Road West, Westport, CT 06881
An imprint of Greenwood Publishing Group, Inc.
www.praeger.com

Printed in the United States of America

The paper used in this book complies with the
Permanent Paper Standard issued by the National
Information Standards Organization (Z39.48–1984).

10 9 8 7 6 5 4 3 2 1

For Alan

Contents

Acknowledgments   ix

Introduction   xi

PART I
Basic Things to Know   1
    1 What Is a Genetics Doctor?   3
    2 Primer on Family History   11
    3 Who Is Affected by Genetic Disease?   21
    4 DNA, Chromosomes, and Genes   31

PART II
Pregnancy and Pregnancy Planning   39
    5 Forewarned and Forearmed   41
    6 When Genetic Disease Runs in a Family   51
    7 Hidden Genetic Risks   67
    8 Prenatal Testing   73
    9 What If a Test Is Positive?   81

PART III
Genetics in Infancy and Childhood   87
    10 Abnormalities in the Fetus and Infant   89

viii CONTENTS

11 Abnormalities in the Child   101
12 When the Problem Cannot Be Fixed   111

PART IV
Genetics in Puberty and Adolescence   119
13 When Things Go Right   121
14 When Things Go Wrong—Female   131
15 When Things Go Wrong—Male   139
16 Teenage Angst   145

PART V
Adult Genetic Disease   151
17 Genetic Conditions That Come on Later   153
18 Genetics of Common Adult Diseases   159
19 Knowledge Is Power   165

APPENDICES   171
Appendix A: Models of Genetic Risk   173
Appendix B: Influences on Dominant
    Genetic Conditions   179

Notes   183

Glossary   187

Index   203

Acknowledgments

Thanks go to Mr. Richard Noyes, the high school teacher who introduced me to genetics—the coolest thing I had ever seen—and to Dr. Larry Jones for just assuming I could learn it. My gratitude as well to Dr. Frank Greenberg, mentor and role model, for showing me the best way to practice it.

The author would also like to thank the following people who were kind enough to read, comment, and encourage: Dr. Stephen Jones, Dr. Elizabeth Purcell-Keith, Mrs. Dawn Scheuerle, Esq., and Dr. Ellen Sher. I am also grateful for the help from the librarians at Planned Parenthood Federation of America and fellow members of the Organization of Teratogen Information Services Listserve for helping me find needed information. Members of the University of the South Alumni Listserve are appreciated for their ideas about what topics are important to educated people who just did not have time to take genetics their junior year.

Introduction

How do we experience genetics in our everyday lives? There are announcements about new discoveries in the paper or on the radio. We get into debates about genetically modified food and human cloning. Or someone in our family is diagnosed with a birth defect or genetic disease.

Most books or classes about genetics start with the basics and move forward from there. Such a strategy is useful in school, but school and life are different things. This book aims to cover the same information but in a way that reflects how most people have their first brush with genetics: when a disease is diagnosed in your family.

Outside of school, you are more likely to encounter genetics in a doctor's office than in a laboratory. But what does that mean? The first part of this book describes the different professionals you are likely to meet in a genetics clinic, explains the information they gather, and gives an overview of some tricky concepts. It also includes a chapter on the basics of DNA and chromosomes. The second part focuses on pregnancy and prenatal diagnosis. Parts three, four, and five discuss genetic problems and birth defects as they affect children, teens, and adults, respectively.

The last chapter of each section I have devoted to some other considerations. These matters are tangential to genetics but are very much a part of patients' lives. Some of these are ethical issues, such as when to involve a teenager in medical decision making. Others are strictly legal definitions or food for thought. I do not presume to be an expert in psychology or law, and readers who would like more information in these areas are encouraged to seek out advice from their own physician, lawyer, or other counselor.

In my own discussions with patients, I try to uphold two principles: (1) information itself is valueless—neither good nor bad; and (2) the only bad decision is the uninformed decision. May this book help you toward making good decisions.

PART I

Basic Things to Know

1 | What Is a Genetics Doctor?

So, you've been referred to a clinical geneticist. What sort of doctor will you see? The geneticists you read about in the paper or see on television are usually laboratory scientists rather than clinical doctors. Your primary care physician has explained that a geneticist can assist you, but exactly who is this person?

GENETICS PHYSICIANS

Doctors who practice genetics have been around for a long time. Historically, they are doctors who have had an interest in inherited diseases or birth defects, so they informally focused their practice in these areas. Remember that it has only been within the last one hundred years that medical specialties as we know them came into being. Before then, a physician's "specialty" was dictated by a particular interest or local need rather than by the area of formal schooling. The most obvious specialties formed first: surgery and obstetrics became separate from general medicine, for example.

In the second half of the 1900s, as our understanding of genetics increased, genetic training became more formal. At that point, doctors who had completed training in a wider field pursued and received more training specifically in genetics. This early instruction tended to be a type of apprenticeship. These doctors would then practice genetics as a subspecialty within the context of their primary specialty.

In 1981 the American Board of Medical Genetics was formed. This board monitors and regulates genetics training and administers certification tests. In 1991 genetics was given the status of a full medical specialty on par with others such as internal medicine, pediatrics, surgery, and ophthalmology. Because genetics deals with the "not normal," the residency training is combined with a primary care specialty—pediatrics, obstetrics and gynecology, or internal medicine. Over the course of four or five years, a doctor receives training in both specialties. That doctor must then pass tests and maintain skills in both specialties.[1]

Clinical geneticists are physicians with an MD or DO degree. They are different from genetic counselors, who have a specialized master's degree (MGC). Some clinical geneticists are trained in more than one aspect of genetics and may direct a diagnostic laboratory, or they may even run a research laboratory. The majority of genetics physicians are pediatricians, but some are obstetricians, internists, or pathologists.

Genetics is now becoming so involved that genetics doctors are subspecializing—seeing a particular set of patients within the larger context of genetics. A pediatric geneticist will concentrate on birth defects and genetic diseases that show up in children. Obstetric geneticists probably do detailed prenatal testing and counseling when a problem is found. They may also do preimplantation diagnosis testing or help women who themselves have genetic diseases. Genetic internists may work with genetic diseases that come on in adulthood or with common diseases with a genetic component, such as high cholesterol or diabetes. Some genetic internists deal with cancer. Others care for people who have survived childhood with a birth defect or genetic disease and have now outgrown their pediatricians.

Patients are referred to a genetics physician or counselor because their problem is thought to have a significant genetic component or to be the result of a problem in fetal development. Table 1.1 shows some reasons for referral. Most commonly, patients are referred to a clinical geneticist by another physician. Children may be referred by their school or foster care program. And certainly, as with all other doctors, patients may come to a geneticist of their own accord because of a specific concern.

The majority of geneticists work at medical schools, but a growing number are in private practice either individually or as part of a multispecialty group. As of 2002 there were 1,075 medical doctors certified in clinical genetics in the United States. Additionally, there were 151 persons with a PhD who were certified to see and counsel patients and 1,410 genetic counselors. Some of these people also hold certification in other areas of genetics, indicating that they received training and passed tests in at least one additional genetics field.

Table 1.1   Possible Reasons for a Genetics Consultation

Obstetric:	Woman with recurrent miscarriages or stillbirths
	Woman or man as part of an infertility evaluation
	Pregnant woman after an abnormal test of the fetus
	Couple if either member has a genetic or heritable condition
Pediatric:	Family history of a genetic or heritable condition
	Pregnant woman with an abnormality in the fetus
	Fetus miscarried/stillborn with a birth defect
	Infant with a birth defect
	Infant with a metabolic problem
	Family history of early infant deaths
Adult:	Diagnosis of a late-onset genetic condition
	Counseling and testing of a late-onset condition
	Family history of a "common" disease
	Extremely high cholesterol
	Early-onset dementia
	Cancer, particularly if early, multifocal, or otherwise unusual

THE GENETICS CLINIC VISIT

In practice, a visit to a geneticist is no different from any other doctor visit. You may be called and asked for some information ahead of time or be asked to bring family photos and to research your family history. The biggest difference you will see is likely to be the level of detail. The genetic interview includes an in-depth family history. You are probably used to telling what caused your parents' or grandparents' deaths. A clinical geneticist will want much more. This is discussed in Chapter 2. If the problem in question is a birth defect or mental retardation in your child, there will be questions about the pregnancy and the time around conception.

The genetics physical exam is not unusual except for the measurements taken. In addition to height, weight, and head circumference, common measurements include hand and foot length, arm span, ear length, distance apart of the eyes, and chest circumference. Other measurements may be done depending upon the problem under consideration. Clinical geneticists examining a child may ask who else in the family has particular features. They may also want to examine one or both parents or a sibling. Many clinical geneticists, particularly those dealing with birth defects and syndromes, will take photographs because, in this business, a picture really is worth a thousand words. If photographs are to be taken, you will be asked to sign a permission form.

Tests done by a clinical geneticist are most frequently blood tests. Occasionally, a test is done on a small piece of skin or other tissue. If any tests are needed, the details will be explained to you during the clinic visit. The clinical geneticist may suggest tests that are familiar, such as X rays and ultrasounds, or may want unusual tests done on common samples. For example, a blood sample, a familiar thing, may be tested for DNA methylation patterns (a way to see whether genes are turned on or off), an unusual test.

Tests for genetic disease are developed first in research labs and then moved to clinical or "diagnostic" labs. Diagnostic labs must maintain quality control procedures not required of research labs and will only offer tests that have recognized usefulness and documented sensitivity and specificity. Diagnostic labs obtain and hold accreditation established by the Clinical Laboratory Improvement Amendments (CLIA), which certify that the labs meet specific professional and functional standards. This allows the labs to release test results to patients.

After the history and physical exam, and after any test results are back, you will receive as much information as is available. This is best done at a second in-person visit. Increasingly, clinical geneticists can give a specific diagnosis. There may be treatment options available, although not always. You will also receive counseling about what can be expected with the condition, what might be helpful at a child's school or in planning for the future, and what the chance is that this same condition will occur again in the family. The more common, or more classic, genetic risk predictions are dealt with in the following chapters.

There are some things that clinical geneticists cannot do. They cannot examine a child and say that the child is guaranteed to be genetically normal. They cannot predict future development, behavior, or illness any better than a child's pediatrician (or grandmother). A clinical geneticist may offer possibilities based on knowledge of a particular condition, but those will be generalizations about the condition more than specific information about you or your child. And a clinical geneticist will not tell you whether or not you should have children or make other specific life decisions: he or she will give you all the information you may need to balance risk and choices, but the final decision about your family structure and life choices is up to you.

As of this writing, all major insurance companies, including Medicaid, cover genetic services—doctor visits and testing. As with any medical situation, it is always a good idea to check with your insurance company about their coverage and your particular plan. Because of discrimination concerns, some patients prefer to pay for the clinic visit and testing themselves. A clinic visit to a genetics doctor may cost a few hundred dollars. Costs for testing varies but can range from $50 to $2,000 depending upon the test. If your insurance plan covers genetic clinic visits and testing, your out-of-pocket costs will be the same as for any other medical specialist.

DISEASE INFORMATION ON THE INTERNET

Seventy percent of medical information on the Internet is wrong or outdated. It is common now for patients to research problems themselves, and the Internet is both useful and fraught with problems. There are two facts to be remembered.

First, stick to the big, well-established sites: the March of Dimes, the National Organization for Rare Disorders, the specific disease support group website. These pages are most likely to have updated, correct information that is free from bias. It must be remembered that these sites have to be useful to anyone who may use them. This means that there are long lists of symptoms and problems for each condition. These lists usually contain anything that has ever happened to anyone with the diagnosis. I caution patients and parents not to read such lists and assume that all these things are relevant to their family. Pick and choose what applies.

Second, list servers and chat groups can be very helpful. However, the anecdotes and comments that are shared lean toward the negative. People complain about their situation, their doctor, their insurance company, and so on. There are a few reason for this. One is that patients and families with more complicated cases are more likely to use the chat rooms. They have more things going on, so they have more things to think and talk about. Another is that the chat groups and list servers can serve a sort of "group therapy" function. They tend to be useful for people to vent their frustrations. People who are doing well are less likely to spend their time typing on their computers. Thus, the discussions are skewed and are not representative of the "average" experience.

GENETIC RESEARCH STUDIES

During your genetics clinic visit, you may be approached about participating in a research study, of which there are thousands. Some people are not comfortable participating in studies, whether they are simple, like answering a few questions, or more complex, like helping test a new drug. That is fine. You will never be "punished" for not participating in a study; you will receive the same care that is otherwise available.

If you choose to participate, you will be helping others even if you get no direct benefit. Remember that information and treatment are available to you because others gave a blood sample or kept a diet diary or took a test. Many studies can be carried out using information in your medical chart or blood samples that you have given for other reasons, so there is no extra burden to you. You do not have to pay to participate in a study, but there may be some small expenses, such as parking. Insurance companies are not informed of a person's participation in a study, although, under some circumstances, they may be petitioned to pay for a medication or cover some other expense.

Some tests that are new or that are for rare diseases may remain in the research lab for a long time. They may not be available to you unless you are part of a study. Historically, research labs would share test results with their study subjects. In the 1990s this practice was made illegal because of quality control concerns, although it still took place under the table. Since 2000 there has been increased emphasis on patient privacy and segregating research from patient care. This has effectively ended the informal practice of releasing research study results to individual patients.

If you agree to participate in a research study, it is important to understand that you will probably not learn the test results. If the research lab has obtained CLIA certification, as mentioned above, you may have legal access to your results, although the burden may be upon you to contact one of the researchers and inquire. It is important to understand that obtaining and maintaining CLIA certification is a bureaucratic and financial burden to labs, so that most research labs will not have CLIA certification. Also, research labs that straddle this line—do research but have CLIA certification—may charge a fee for some or all of the sample processing.

Whatever the study, it is your right to know the risks and benefits. Giving "informed consent" does not just mean signing a piece of paper. It means understanding to the best of your ability what is happening. Table 1.2 lists some questions you can ask if you are approached about participating in a study. The person explaining the study should be able to answer all these questions—and any others you may have—to your satisfaction. If they are not, and you are interested in the study, ask to speak to another researcher before consenting to participate.

Table 1.2   Questions to Ask When Considering a Genetic Research Study

Financial disclosure
   Who is doing the study?
   Who is paying for the study?
   Will there be any charge to my insurance company?

Goals of the study
   What does the study test?
   Is this a long-term or a short-term project?
   Can I have a copy of any papers already written?
   How will the results of the study be reported?
   Will I get to know my own results?

Logistics
   What do I have to do?
   How many times do I have to do it?
   Will I have to come back or do something over time?
   Will I be admitted to the hospital for testing?
   Will I be reimbursed for parking and other expenses?
   Will the study arrange with my work/school for me to be absent?

Study subject rights
   How will the study differ from routine care/treatment?
   What are the risks of the study?
   What are the potential benefits of the study to me? To others?
   What happens if I get sick during the study?
   What if a problem occurs during the study?
   Can I drop out at any time?
   If I've given a sample, how can I get it back if I drop out?
   Will my sample be used for studies other than this one?
      If so, will I be contacted beforehand?

Some groups of people are concerned about medical research in general, and genetic research in particular, because of historic study subject abuse. Because of that history, research involving human subjects is overseen by review boards and committees that require all research protocols to protect their participants. Even with these protections, some minority groups are understandably distrustful when approached about studies and choose not to participate. The unfortunate result is that diagnostic tests and treatments most helpful to these groups will be delayed. If you have concerns about genetic research because of your race, ethnicity, age, sex, socioeconomic status, or something else, please discuss this with the researcher. The people most assisted by your participation are people just like you.

THE BIG PICTURE

Unlike other branches of medicine, genetics has developed a mystique. Some of this is understandable: genetics addresses health and illness at a level not previously available. On the other hand, genetics is not magic. It is just a tool. Genetics does not change the general aspects of medicine, it just expands them. For example, it was possible one hundred years ago to estimate someone's life span based upon the longevity of the parents or to predict the health and normality of a baby based upon the family and its environment. The idea of making predictions is not different. All genetics has done has improved, or at least formalized, our ability to predict.

So, you've been referred to a clinical geneticist. It is disturbing enough to have to see a specialist when a problem suddenly is found or suspected, but the mystique surrounding genetics makes this referral doubly uncomfortable. There is, however, nothing mysterious about genetics. In some ways it is more scientific than other branches of medicine. In other ways it is more about the "art" part of medicine. Whatever the reason for the visit, it will be about telling and receiving information, learning what decisions may need to be made, and realizing that you are not as alone in your situation as you may think.

2 Primer on Family History

Some of the first comments made about a newborn child are "She has her dad's nose," or "He has gramma's chin." Fanciful or factual, we all recognize that children inherit their family's characteristics. Sometimes the family has something unusual about it that affects more than one member. Communities have recognized forever that some traits "run" in families or happen more frequently under some circumstances.

BASIC TERMS

Human beings have understood genetic inheritance for millennia in an informal way. We know this because historic and current human cultures proscribe marriage and reproduction based upon some idea that disease is heritable. Many, perhaps most, of these laws were in place before there was any basic science understanding of genetics. Marriages between full siblings, for example, are illegal/taboo everywhere these days. Those cultures that support intrafamilial marriages have specific rules governing how closely related by blood a couple may be. There are some old wives' tales that have sprung up about consanguinity (having children with someone to whom you are genetically related) that are probably an effect of the cultural taboos. In some cases, specific heritability of disease was recognized a long time ago. The Talmud has an exemption from circumcision when there is a maternal family history of bleeding.[1] The early Hebrews had observed the disease we now know as hemophilia and had devised a way to deal with it. Even without understanding the biochemistry or knowing the gene, they could predict that a problem might happen. And, while it has been bastardized by the social Darwinism movements, it is generally true that short, pretty, or physically talented parents tend to beget short, pretty, or physically talented children.

Table 2.1 defines some useful terms. Some conditions are *genetic* without being *heritable* or *familial*. Other conditions are *congenital* but not genetic. For example, trisomy 21 (Down syndrome) is genetic—it is caused by a chromosome abnormality—but 90% of the cases result from a de novo change in the genetic material. The condition is unique to the one affected person in the family. These cases are not heritable and are not familial. It is unlikely that others in the family are at higher risk of having a child with trisomy 21 because the one child was born with it.

Fetal alcohol syndrome (FAS) is *congenital* because it is present from birth, but not genetic. It is caused by in utero exposure to alcohol. FAS is an environmental condition because it is the result of an intrauterine environment that did not support normal fetal growth and development. On the other hand, FAS may be *familial* if the mother has other children similarly affected or if other women in the family are unable to curb their alcohol intake during pregnancy.

Table 2.1   Definitions

Birth defect: Also called a "congenital anomaly." An abnormality in physical structure that is present at birth. This can be major, like a missing limb, or minor, like a skin tag in front of the ear. Can be genetic or environmental. Can be familial.

Congenital: Present at birth. May be diagnosed by prenatal ultrasound, or may not be discovered until later in life. Can be genetic or environmental. Can be familial.

Familial: Affecting more than one member of the family. Can be genetic or environmental. Can be congenital or late-onset.

Genetic: Caused by a change in the structure of DNA. This may be a small change, such as a single base pair mutation, or a big change, such as an entire missing or extra chromosome. It may be a change in the nuclear (cellular) DNA or in the mitochondrial DNA. Not all genetic conditions are heritable or familial, although most are.

Heritable: Capable of being passed from parent to child. Usually genetic. Can be congenital or late-onset.

Late-onset: Conditions manifesting later in life. Can be genetic or environmental. Can be heritable.

The term "congenital" is problematic. Most correctly it means "present at birth," and indeed, a syndrome or birth defect may be obvious in the delivery room. However, a condition may show symptoms from birth but because they are so subtle the diagnosis is not made until later. Some conditions diagnosed later in infancy or childhood may not have been apparent earlier. In these cases, the condition is said to have infantile or childhood onset with the understanding that the underlying problem predates that. There may even have been a birth defect that was present at birth but was never noticed. For example, a child may be born with only one kidney, but if that child is otherwise healthy, there is no reason to look for a problem. The lack of a kidney may go unnoticed for years until there is a reason to do the X ray or ultrasound that reveals the birth defect.

Conditions are said to be "late-onset" if the symptoms do not manifest until adulthood. A late-onset condition can be genetic and/or familial. It can be inherited and may be passed on to children. Huntington disease is the paradigm late-onset genetic condition (although the youngest patient diagnosed to date is 2 years). It is genetic—resulting from a change in the gene—both heritable and familial and usually comes on after the age of 30. Technically, the genetic change that causes Huntington disease is congenital: the mutation is present since before birth. The disease symptoms themselves are late-onset.

In practice these terms are used rather loosely, but it is important to understand at the very least that "genetic," "congenital," and "familial" are not synonymous. It also must be understood that the line between a genetic condition and an environmental condition is not distinct. There are some conditions that are clearly and only genetic, such as achondroplasia or trisomy 21. There are others that are only environmental, such as concussion and amputation. Everything else is somewhere in the middle. Even FAS is not cleanly environmental, as its presence and severity depend upon such things as a baby's genetic susceptibility and a mother's ability to metabolize alcohol.

RELATIONSHIPS

Family relationship and health are significant to one's genetics, and the family history is an important part of a genetic evaluation. The genetic family history is more detailed than a routine genealogy. It is also more involved than the family history typically taken by other doctors. The detail to which a geneticist will take a family history depends on the problem being presented.

The person with the condition in question is called the proband. (If the person seeking genetic consultation is healthy, she may instead be called a consultand.) Family members are then ranked into primary, or first-degree, relatives, second-degree relatives, and so forth (Table 2.2). The degree translates into genetic relatedness. Primary relatives are parents, siblings, and children of the proband—people who share on average 1/2 of their genetic material with the proband. Secondary relatives are the next step out and share 1/4 of their genetic material—grandparents, aunts/uncles, grandchildren. Tertiary relatives share 1/8 of the genetic material and are first cousins, great grandparents, great grandchildren.

There are many details to a genetic family history that seem so logical after the fact but can be difficult to organize beforehand. Take the issue of cousins. What really is the difference between a second cousin and a first cousin once removed? There is a standard definition. Figure 2.1 will be helpful. First cousins are children of siblings: a brother's child and his sister's child are first cousins. Second cousins are first cousins' children. Third cousins are the children of second cousins, and so forth. A cousin is "removed" by generation. Cousins who are one generation apart are once removed, those who are two generations apart are twice removed, and so on. By convention, the higher generation is used as the starting point. When referring to two cousins as "removed"—first cousins once removed—"first cousins" is the highest level on the pedigree. Since they are "removed" they are, by definition, in different generations.

Looking at Figure 2.1, part B, there are four relationships demonstrated. Relationship $\mathbb{A}$ is indicated for orientation sake: it is a typical aunt/niece set. A woman and her brother's daughter are aunt and niece. Relationships $\mathbb{B}$ and $\mathbb{D}$ are both "once removed." In $\mathbb{B}$, the higher of the two is on the first cousin level. Thus, the $\mathbb{B}$ relationship is first cousins once removed. It is very similar in $\mathbb{D}$, except for the generations involved. In this case, the higher cousin in the pedigree is in the second cousin generation. Thus, the $\mathbb{D}$ relationship is second cousins once removed. In relationship $\mathbb{C}$, the higher person is in the first cousin generation, but the indicated relatives

Table 2.2   Genetic Relatedness in a Family History

Primary relatives: Share 1/2 of their genetic material with the proband
  Parents, children, siblings

Secondary relatives: Share 1/4 of their genetic material with the proband
  Grandparents, grandchildren, aunts, uncles

Tertiary relatives: Share 1/8 of their genetic material with the proband
  Great grandparents, great grandchildren, first cousins

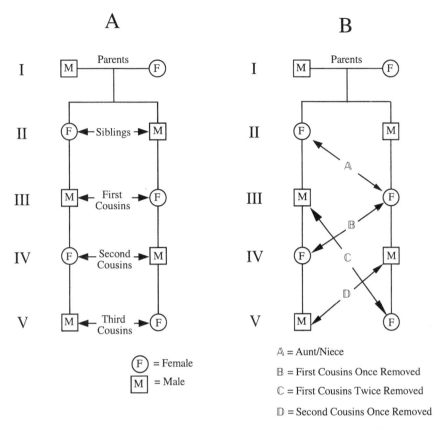

A

B

Figure 2.1 Cousins—first, second, third, and so on, and "removed" (spouses are left out for simplicity).

are two generations apart: the male is in the same generation as the female's grandmother. So, these two people are first cousins twice removed.

CONSTRUCTING PEDIGREES

Geneticists use a pictorial representation of the family that helps clarify relationships. Figures 2.2 and 2.3 show the various symbols used and a standard family pedigree—sometimes called a genogram. Circles represent females, squares represent males, and diamonds represent persons of unknown sex. The circles, squares, and diamonds are arranged in a standard fashion and are filled in to represent that the person is affected by a given condition. Now it is easier to see the widening circles of relatedness. It is also a much simpler matter to trace a heritable problem

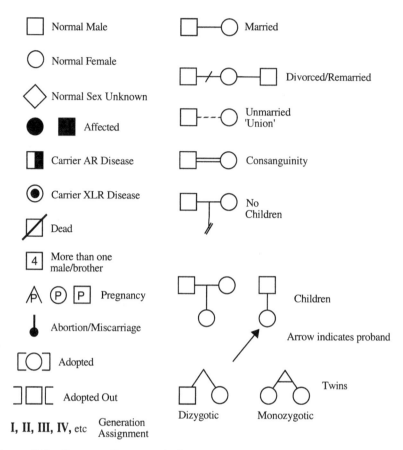

Figure 2.2 Some pedigree symbols.

through a family or to see a pattern that previously was missed. Pedigrees will be used in the following chapters to illustrate patterns of inheritance.

The pedigree in Figure 2.3 shows a typical family. The following paragraph describes the family in narrative for comparison with the figure. Initially, the narrative will make more sense because it is a familiar form. It is, however, easy to see that the paragraph is more laborious than the picture, and this is a simple family. In a complex family with more people, significant genetic disease, a higher number of divorces and remarriages, and so on, it would become impossible to tease information out of a narrative. Genetic pedigrees relieve most of the tedium and make the information much more accessible.

There are two parents, mother, Amanda, age 35, and father, José, age 38, and two full siblings, a boy, John, age 14, and a girl, Anika, age 11.

Anika is the proband. She has spina bifida. The mother also had a sponta-neous abortion at 15 weeks in her first pregnancy. The sex of that preg-nancy is unknown. The parents are divorced and the mother has remarried. The mother has a child in her new marriage. That child is a girl, Mary, age 3. José, the father, lost a finger in a work accident. The father's father, Emmanuel, is deceased because of a stroke at age 88. His family name is Treviño and he was born in San Salvador. His family is mostly Mayan. The father's mother, Josephine, is alive at age 79 and is healthy except for arthritis and hearing loss. Her family name is Suarez and she comes from Nicaragua. Her ethnic group is only listed as "Hispanic." The father has a brother, Gomez, who is 40 and has three children, two daughters, Sasha, age 15, and Margaret, age 10, and a son, Isaac, age 12. The mother's par-ents are both deceased. Her father, Charles, died at age 51 in an automo-bile accident. He had been born with a cleft lip. His family name was O'Malley and he was Irish. Her mother, Farah, died at age 60 of breast cancer. Her family name was Gallieni and she was part Italian and part Ethiopian. The mother has a sister, Elana, age 32, who has one child, a girl named Roma, age 8. Roma was born with a cleft lip.

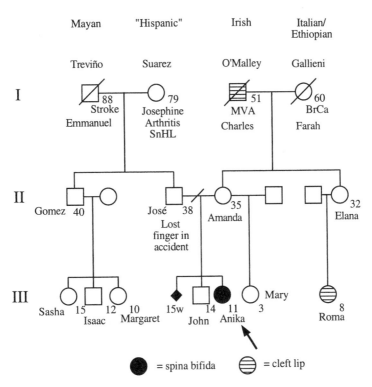

Figure 2.3 Standard simple pedigree.

One thing immediately apparent is how much easier the two cleft lip patients are to find in the picture. It is also much more obvious how they are related. This sort of knowledge—who is affected and how they are related—helps the geneticist predict the risk of similar problems in other relatives. Pedigrees can also be used to list results of genetic tests or other information that contributes to the calculation of risk.

IMPORTANT FAMILY HISTORY INFORMATION

During the clinic visit, the family history is taken, and the pedigree constructed, as part of the regular medical interview process. Geneticists will draw out the pedigree as part of note taking and will ask questions in a particular pattern. Table 2.3 suggests some investigation that can be done before the clinic visit to give a genetic family history. Information about each person, including name, age or year of birth, whether they are living or dead, health status or cause of death, ethnicity and national origin, will be asked. It is important to note whether someone was adopted and what, if any, genetic relationship there may be with the rest of the family. With the increased use of artificial reproductive technology, it is important to know whether a child conceived by in vitro fertilization (IVF) is biologically related to the parents. All of these pieces of data help paint the picture of individual and general family health and longevity. Race, ethnicity, and place of origin are collected because some

Table 2.3   Preparing for a Genetic Family History—Things to Know

---

Any birth defects or genetic conditions in the family

Miscarriages and stillbirths

Ages and causes of death of any child who died in infancy or childhood

Any relative with mental retardation, developmental problems, or significant sight/hearing loss

Names and years of birth (or age) of as many relatives as possible, including cousins

Major health problems and/or surgeries

Causes of death for adults

Last names of grandparents, their ethnic groups, and their places of origin
    Note: North America as a place of origin is only true for Native Americans

Differentiate full siblings from half or step siblings and adopted children

Family photos are also extremely helpful to the geneticist

---

birth defects and genetic conditions vary in incidence among races. Place of origin is asked as a way to determine whether there are blood relations between married individuals. If a husband and wife believe they have no relatives in common but both come from the same small town, there is a chance that they are genetically related.

The geneticist will also candidly ask an unexpected question of any consulting parents: "Is there any chance you are related by blood?" As with asking place of origin, the geneticist is attempting to determine consanguinity—the likelihood that both members of a couple share genetic traits—which increases the risk of problems in children. In the exam room, the question is most often answered with laughter. The geneticist is not questioning to criticize or challenge: in some cultures it is perfectly acceptable that one's spouse is a cousin or other known relation. (Persons from such cultures usually give exquisite family histories because their traditions are family- or clan-oriented and they know information in great detail.) Unfortunately, asking this question rarely turns up cases of incest, which is extremely important to know for many reasons, not the least of which are genetic and legal.

You will note that the genetic family history incorporates information about abortions[2] and stillbirths. These are included because repeated loss of pregnancy is associated with both maternal health and some genetic conditions. In fact, repeated pregnancy loss can be the primary purpose of referral to a geneticist. Spontaneous abortions—miscarriages—are very common but they are not typically discussed, even within a family. A woman may have had one or more spontaneous abortions without her own children knowing. Elective abortions may have been done on medical grounds or because of a birth defect in a previous pregnancy, which is obviously significant.

Knowing about children who died in infancy or childhood is extremely important, particularly in cases of birth defects and congenital disease. Since the invention of antibiotics, fewer children die of infectious disease. Genetics and birth defects are now the leading cause of infant death in the developed world.[3] If there is a family history of infant or childhood death, even unexplained, the geneticist needs to know about it. As with repeated pregnancy loss, one or more children who died in the first few years of life can indicate a genetic disease in the family.

THINKING ABOUT FAMILY HISTORY

Recent advances in genetic science have emphasized that each patient should be considered in the context of the family. This is not really a new concept, although it does get treated as such. Family genetics and environment have always been important. Now they are important in a more formal way. In thinking about a genetics consultation or clinic visit, the best preparation is a review of the patient's family history. Often persons do not know small details that may be important or the health problems of a family member that turn out to be relevant.

In the case of an adult patient, the family history covers both past and future generations. Although it is called a "history," the family does include children, grandchildren, and current pregnancies. There are some genetic conditions that worsen as they are passed from generation to generation. The diagnosis of a genetic condition in a grandchild may give clues to the appropriate diagnosis in the grandmother. Also, conditions and physical features change with age. Since many conditions are classically described in children, the features may be different, more subtle, or gone altogether in adults. Thinking of the patient and family as a continuum leads to both better care of the patient and advances in understanding of disease.

3 Who Is Affected by Genetic Disease?

Before germs were discovered in the late 1800s, disease was attributed to many things: bad air, evil spirits, punishments from God, and so on. Once the germ theory of disease was established, bacteria and viruses were identified and useful antibiotics and vaccines were invented. Today we understand the basis of infection so well that germs are only occasionally scary and, despite admonitions to bundle up, mothers really do know that colds are caused by viruses and not by wet feet. Infections are still common, but they do not seem so because we have become so good at curing or controlling them. Certainly there are some exceptions— malaria, HIV, SARS—but even those that do not have a cure can be managed. If there is no treatment, our knowledge about the germs allows us to invent prevention strategies.

THE SPECTRUM OF GENETIC DISEASE

Genetics is as ubiquitous as infection as a contributor to human disease. In Chapter 2 there was a brief discussion about genetic versus environmental conditions. Here we can take it further. It has been recognized for a long time that there is a genetic contribution to birth defects such as cleft lip, spina bifida, and club feet. It has quickly become apparent that common adult conditions such as heart disease, high blood pressure, and dementia also have a genetic component.

Figure 3.1 shows the spectrum of disease as it relates to genetics. The

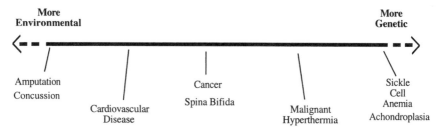

Figure 3.1   The spectrum of human disease and its causes. Other things that fall in the middle part of the spectrum are allergies, cleft lip, club foot, dementia, diabetes, emphysema, infertility, infectious disease, kidney failure, mental retardation, schizophrenia, seizures, wound healing, and most other conditions in which the body changes or responds to something.

items on the far right are purely genetic. Those on the far left are purely acquired or environmental. Everything in between is caused by some combination of the two. In some cases, a condition will not happen because the environmental insult is not present: a person with no access to alcohol will not develop alcoholic liver cirrhosis, even if there is a high genetic risk. Other conditions are avoided because there is no genetic susceptibility, even if the environment is harmful: some rare persons do not get lung cancer even though they smoke for most of their lives.

This type of condition—all the stuff in the middle of the spectrum—is called *multifactorial* because it arises only when a combination of circumstances are present. It is exactly what it sounds like: there are many factors that play into the condition. There is no single cause. Genetics plays a role, so there are genes involved, but environment and chance also contribute. If just a few genes are involved, the condition is oligogenic. If there are many genes, it is polygenic. Furthermore, each gene may contribute to a different degree or a gene may be detrimental only if another specific gene is mutated.

This chapter will concentrate on the genetic contribution to disease. Environmental risks are covered in other works and can be difficult to discuss. There are some environmental exposures that are accepted as causing disease: smoking and lung cancer/emphysema, alcohol use in pregnancy and mental retardation in the offspring, recurrent concussion and neurologic dysfunction (Table 3.1). True environmental exposure is hard to measure. This becomes more difficult when the problem in question is a birth defect and exposure to the fetus depends upon the way mom's body metabolizes something.

Table 3.1 Environmental Factors That Contribute to Multifactorial Conditions

Environmental Factor	Related Multifactorial Condition
Cigarette Smoking	Lung cancer, emphysema, heart disease
Air Pollution	Asthma
Folic Acid Deficiency	Spina Bifida in child, heart disease, stroke
Concussion	Parkinson Disease
Alcohol	Liver cirrhosis
Asbestos	Asbestosis - a lung disease
Lead	Growth problems and mental retardation

TWO DIFFICULT CONCEPTS

There are two difficult concepts to be mastered in discussions of genetics, which are most apparent in multifactorial conditions. The first is the concept of statistical risk. The second is the concept of what genes are present in which persons.

Statistical Risk

If statistics were understood, no one would buy lottery tickets and everyone would be comfortable flying in airplanes. Statistical risk, the chance that a particular thing will happen, is a difficult concept. There are two basic ways to think about risk. One way is that risk is based upon a specific mathematical calculation, like the lottery. The "risk" of winning the lottery is very precisely calculated based upon the chance that given numbers will be randomly chosen. If it is a three-pick lottery with each pick being of numbers 1 to 50, the chance of a specific combination is as follows (see Figure 3.2):

$$6 \times (1/50 \times 1/49 \times 1/48) = 1/19,600.$$

In a six-pick lottery, the chance is

$$720 \times (1/50 \times 1/49 \times 1/48 \times 1/47 \times 1/46 \times 1/45) = 1/15,890,700.$$

This "risk" can be precisely and accurately calculated because it is based upon mathematical constants. The chance of winning does not change with the number of tickets sold.

Other risk is based upon historical observations of the population or of a particular situation. In this case the numbers are more of a guide than an absolute. The risk of injury or death in the decade 1987 to 1996 in an

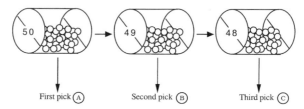

First pick (A)   Second pick (B)   Third pick (C)

The lottery starts with 50 balls in a barrel. After one is picked there are 49 in the barrel. After two are picked there are 48, etc.

Three Pick Lottery:

The chance that ball A is one of your numbers is 3 chances in 50 balls.
The chance that ball B is one of your numbers is 2 in 49. The chance that ball C is your remaining number is 1 in 48.

So, the chance that all three of your numbers are picked is 3/50 x 2/49 x 1/48 = 6 x (1/50 x 1/49 x 1/48) = 1/19,600.

Six Pick Lottery:

The chance that all six numbers are picked is
      6/50 x 5/49 x 4/48 x 3/47 x 2/46 x 1/45 = 720 x (1/50 x 1/49 x 1/48 x 1/47 x 1/46 x 1/45) = 15,890,700.

Figure 3.2 The statistics of a lottery. There are 50 lottery balls, numbered 1 through 50.

aviation accident was 1/7,000,000 persons.[1] One other interpretation of these data says that one person, flying every single day, risks dying once every 19,000 years.[2] What are these numbers really measuring? They are measuring an observation: of the millions of person/miles flown in the observed decade, x number of people died. It is history. It is useful as a starting point, but is only one of a number of items to be considered when thinking about future risk. Unlike lottery chances, the risk of injury while flying does change over time because it is based upon uncontrollable circumstances that may or may not happen.

Other variables for this particular risk might be: How many people traveled by air? What is the actual number of deaths? What changes have been made to reduce risk since these observations were made? What changes have happened that increase risk? In any one trip by plane, what is the risk of injury or death? How does this compare to other modes of travel? All of these facts, some of them measurable, play into the calculation of risk.

Numbers are easy to read but can be difficult to interpret. The more data that are available, the better the calculation. A patient can be told that there is a 30% risk of developing a condition. That means that, when many people of the same age, sex, family history, health, habits, income, and so on, were compared, one-third of them developed a particular disease. The risk is empiric/observed/historic rather than deduced/calculated. Increasing knowledge about genetics is changing this rough estimate to a degree, but we have a long way to go before an individual's health prediction can be precise. One goal of genetics is to change risk estimates so that they are based upon factors internal to the patient and are, therefore, more relevant to an individual patient.

Who Has What Genes

All tissues of the body, except red blood cells, contain the entire genome, although not all genes are active in all tissues. Human beings all have the same basic genome with some variation. Within our species there are gene variations that are perfectly normal, such as those that cause different skin colors. We also all carry deleterious gene mutations. Some are bad for us and some are bad for our offspring. When the gene is mutated, it only matters in the relevant tissue. A gene mutation that causes problems in the brain does not matter if the mutation is only present in cells of the fingernail bed.

Unfortunately, genes tend to be named, or nicknamed, based upon the disease caused when the gene does not work. So, we refer to the "cystic fibrosis" gene or the "breast cancer" gene as if it is only present when the disease is diagnosed. This is not so. The gene in the normal form is present at all times, has a specific role, and does not contribute to disease. In fact, the normal gene is necessary for standard species function. So, we all have the "breast cancer" gene, BRCA1, but in the vast majority of us, it is normal and contributing to our health rather than to cancer.

MULTIFACTORIAL CONDITIONS

Genes involved in multifactorial conditions are also always present in everyone. There seems to be enough redundancy in the human system that one gene can pick up the slack when another is working at less than full capacity. This is an assumption. We are still very early in understanding how genes and their products work and interact. In a multigene system, it is only when all genes are abnormal, or when one mutated gene overwhelms the others, that the system breaks down. Sometimes all genes can be fine but an environmental contribution, such as smoking or folic acid deficiency, can cause problems for which the genes cannot compensate.

Think of a bag of marbles, as shown in Figure 3.3. Some marbles are black, and those represent genes. Patterned marbles are environmental factors such as smoking or radiation. White marbles represent stochastic factors—chance or influences that are unidentifiable. So, each marble represents a gene or an environmental toxin or luck: the various factors

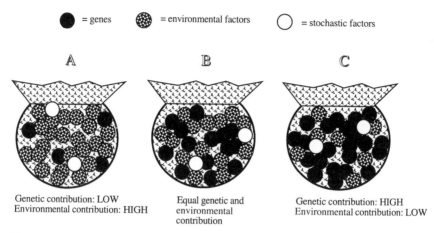

Genetic contribution: LOW
Environmental contribution: HIGH

Equal genetic and
environmental
contribution

Genetic contribution: HIGH
Environmental contribution: LOW

Figure 3.3 Contributions to multifactorial conditions. The factors contributing to disease are represented by marbles. A bag of marbles can be full in many different combinations. Multifactorial disease can be caused by many different combinations of genes, environmental factors, and chance.

that contribute to a multifactorial condition. In Figure 3.3 there are three bags of marbles. They are equally filled, but the combination of marbles in each bag is different. Bag A is filled mostly with patterned marbles, Bag C with black marbles, and Bag B with an equal ratio. All bags have a couple of white marbles representing uncontrollable or unknowable elements.

Multifactorial disease can be thought of the same way. Figure 3.4 shows three persons, A, B, and C, each with the same risk of a condition. In this case let's say they each have a 30% risk of having a heart attack in the next ten years. Person A is at risk because of environmental factors. Person B is at risk because of an equal combination of environmental factors and genetics. Person C has a low environmental contribution but a high genetic risk. All persons are susceptible to the influence of stochastic factors.

However, people do not all have an equal risk of a particular condition. If they did, medicine in general and genetics in particular would not be so complex. The likelihood that someone will have a heart attack or give birth to a baby with a birth defect is different from person to person. There are two models used to discuss the interpersonal variation in disease risk: the Basic Model and the Threshold Model. In some conditions, one model is more useful than the other, although both can be used at some level for anything. These models are described here in a basic fashion. More information can be found in Appendix A.

MODELS OF RISK

The Basic Model can be used to demonstrate or estimate disease risk: the statistical likelihood that someone will be affected with a disease. In the Basic Model, everyone has some degree of risk. Overall risk is distributed so that there are a few people with very low risk, a few people with very high risk, and everyone else in between. Most people have average risk. The risk is never zero, although it can be very low. The risk is never 100% until an actual diagnosis is made.

Using the bag of marbles analogy in the Basic Model, everyone has a bag with some marbles in it and all bags are at risk of breaking. Some people have bags with just a few marbles, so the risk of breakage is low (but not impossible). Others have bags with many marbles, and the risk is high (although not absolute). Most people fall somewhere in the middle, in the normal distribution.

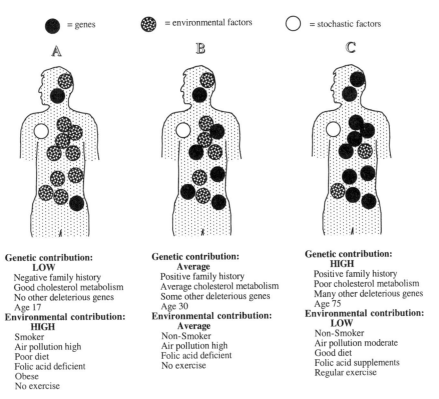

Figure 3.4 Three persons with equal risk of a multifactorial disease, in this case heart disease. Person A's risk is mostly environmental. Person B's risk is equally genetic and environmental. Person C's risk is mostly genetic.

The other model is the Threshold Model. The idea here is that there is no risk at all until a particular degree of liability is reached. Below that threshold, the disease or condition does not occur, regardless of the presence of liability factors. Going back to the bag of marbles, the Threshold Model says that all bags are intact up to a certain point. After that point is reached, all bags break. There is no risk of breakage at all when there are just a few marbles or even an average number of marbles.

Both models are snapshots. Real risk is based upon things that are not constant, such as age or smoking exposure. For an individual, the number and type of marbles in the bag will change over his or her lifetime. Also, this is the risk of a particular thing, such as breast cancer or spina bifida. It is not a global risk of everything. In reality, each person has many bags of marbles, each representing a different disease or condition and each having its own risk of breaking. These risks may be interrelated or they may be independent.

The Basic Model and the Threshold Model are based upon observations. The flow of information is as follows: (1) observation of phenomenon, (2) construction of the measurement/prediction model, (3) use of the model for prediction in other phenomena. It should be remembered that the models are based upon things that manifest in certain ways. A given model may not be useful when the situation is different from the one used to construct the model.

RISK CALCULATIONS

There is a baseline population risk for any disease or condition. That baseline risk is set by observing thousands of people over many years. For example, clinical geneticists will typically quote a risk of 3–5% in any pregnancy for having a baby with a birth defect. In other words, in one hundred healthy pregnancies that carry to term, three, four, or five of those babies will have a significant birth defect. This is total risk. Some of these birth defects will reveal hidden gene mutations in the parents, some will be new mutations or inherited conditions, and some will be multifactorial conditions.

There are four genetic factors that increase someone's risk of being born with or developing a multifactorial condition. These points were originally established by observation of families. If any of these criteria are present, the chance of the condition happening again is higher. These factors are only important in multifactorial conditions. In purely genetic conditions caused by a single gene mutation, risk of recurrence is much more directly determined (see Chapters 6 and 7).

1. Having one or more relatives with the same condition: This indicates that the genetic contribution to the condition is greater. In reality, the risk in the family has not changed, although it seems that way. As more people in the family are affected, there is a better picture of actual risk. Also, as more people are affected, the risk approaches 50%.
2. Being closely related to the affected individual: More closely related persons share more of both their genetics and their environment. Two closely related people are more likely to have inherited the same deleterious gene (see Chapter 2, Relationships).
3. If the proband is of the less frequently affected sex: Some conditions are more common in one sex than the other. For example, cleft lip is more common in males. A newborn is at greater risk of having a cleft lip if the mother (the less common sex) is affected than if the father is. This suggests that the affected individual, and therefore the family, has more genetic liability.
4. If the proband is severely affected: It is observed that the chance of a condition recurring in a family is higher if the first affected person is severely affected. As with (3) above, this suggests that there are more liability factors in the family.

These risk factors are best established for multifactorial birth defects. They are used to predict the chance that the parents will have a second child similarly affected. For unaffected parents, the chance that a child will be born with a cleft lip is about 1 chance in 1,000 (0.1%). After one child is so affected, the risk of recurrence—the probability that the next sibling will have a cleft lip—is 1 in 25 (4%). If a second child has the same condition, then the risk of recurrence in a third child is 1 in 4 (25%). Retrospectively, the risk to the other children was also 25%, but there was no way to know that until enough children were born. There was no clue that the risk was that high.

COMMON THINGS ARE COMMON

The genetics of common disease is important precisely because these conditions affect so many people. Because of the sheer numbers of people involved, it is most likely that advances in genetic diagnosis and treatment will be made in those diseases that are not strictly genetic. The complicating factor is that the more common a condition is, the more numerous the causes of it. That makes it more difficult to find the primary cause of a common condition. It also complicates the ability to predict that such a condition will happen.

4 DNA, Chromosomes, and Genes

Deoxyribonucleic acid (DNA) is our hereditary material. It is the storage medium for information passed from parent to child. DNA was first discovered in 1871, defined as the hereditary material in 1883, and its structure was described in 1953.[1] Today, short descriptions of DNA appear in newspapers and magazines, and high school students learn how to extract it from bananas. While the basic structure of DNA is simple, its functions and interactions are complex. This chapter will review the chemistry of DNA, how it is organized into chromosomes, and how it forms genes.

DNA STRUCTURE

Chemically, DNA is an acid. This does not mean that DNA is corrosive or dangerous, but being an acid does make it interactive with other molecules: it is stable, but it is not inert. Structurally, DNA looks like a ladder—it is often described as a spiral staircase. The rails of the ladder or staircase are chains of alternating sugar and phosphate molecules running in opposite directions. The sugar is deoxyribose. The rungs are the DNA bases, of which there are four: adenine (A), guanine (G), cytosine (C), and thymine (T) (Figure 4.1). Each rung has a pair of bases, one of which is bound to each sugar-phosphate backbone. The opposed bases are chemically charged and are attracted to each other, holding the ladder or staircase together. The two bases in a rung are a "base pair." The

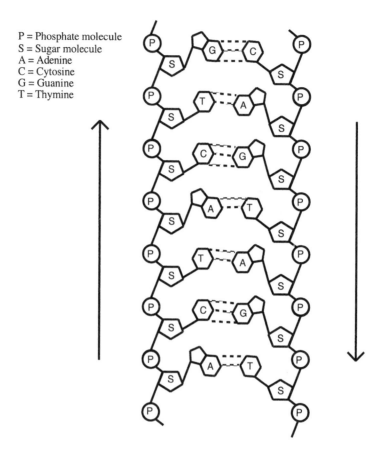

P = Phosphate molecule
S = Sugar molecule
A = Adenine
C = Cytosine
G = Guanine
T = Thymine

Figure 4.1   The structure of DNA.

bases always pair adenine:thymine (A:T) and guanine:cytosine (G:C). More detailed information about the biochemistry of DNA can be found in Appendix B.

DNA is called a double helix: "double" because there are the two sugar-phosphate backbones—two strands—with bases; "helix" because the ladder gently turns—hence the spiral staircase analogy. The elementary shape of DNA is strictly dictated by the various chemical interactions that form the molecule.[2] It can also be thought of as a zipper because that is how DNA works. The two DNA strands must be "unzipped" to expose the bases.

To understand how DNA works in the cell, we must first understand something about proteins. Proteins are also large molecules made up of smaller parts. In proteins those parts, the basic units, are amino acids.

The order of the amino acids in a protein dictates how the protein takes shape and how it carries out its function. The trick is to get from the string of bases in the DNA to the string of amino acids in a protein.

Information is stored in the order of the bases on one side of the double helix. Our language alphabet works the same way: "information" comes from the order of letters in a word. Even though English has only twenty-six letters, it is possible to make an infinite number of words. The bases in DNA work the same way. The helix is unwound and unzipped to expose the bases. The four bases—A, C, G, and T— occur in what appears to be a random pattern, but when read in "triplets," three bases in a row, the cell can decipher the stored information. There are 64 possible triplet combinations of the four bases: ACC, AAA, GAT, TGC, and so on. These triplets are called *codons*. Each codon codes for a particular amino acid. This is the "genetic code": the matching of DNA triplets to specific amino acids. Strings of codons translate into strings of protein amino acids. Thus, a section of DNA that we call a gene instructs the cell to make a particular protein or part of a protein.

There is an intermediate molecule called ribonucleic acid (RNA) that is the processing agent moving information from DNA to protein. RNA is similar to DNA except that it is single stranded, uses ribose instead of deoxyribose, and has uracil (U) instead of thymine. The genetic information is *transcribed* from DNA to RNA and then *translated* from RNA to protein. There are some stretches of DNA that just code for RNA molecules. The RNA, in turn, manages the DNA or runs the mechanics of translating the genetic information from DNA to protein. It has recently been discovered that some RNA strands regulate others and that some proteins interact directly with RNA. These are other ways that the cell manipulates genetic information.

Just to finish out some definitions, since DNA is a double helix it has a built-in template and is self-reproducing (it can make another copy of itself because it has an intrinsic model). When DNA is used to make more DNA, it is said to be *replicated*. Some viruses known as retroviruses (like HIV) can produce DNA from RNA. The process of moving information from RNA back to DNA is *reverse transcription*. It is also possible to have *RNA replication* and there may be *protein replication*. *Reverse translation*— creating RNA from the information in a protein—is theorized but has not been proven.

All of these processes make up the Central Dogma of Biology, which is shown in Figure 4.2. With the addition of new discoveries, it has become a little less dogmatic but a lot more interesting.

WHAT IS A GENE?

The first person to talk about genes was Gregor Mendel (1822–1884), a monk who worked with garden peas. He worked in what is now Brno, in the Czech Republic. He cross-bred the pea plants and was able to observe, describe, and predict the inheritance of characteristics such as flower color, seed shape, and plant height. We still refer to the most common inheritance patterns as Mendelian, and these will be discussed below and in other chapters.

Mendel was either very lucky or very smart—or some combination of the two. He chose plant characteristics that were, genetically, independent of each other. This gave him very clean results.[3] He was able to define a gene rather precisely: a piece of genetic information that operates independently from other pieces, that defines a specific single physical characteristic, and that is inherited in a predictable manner.

Today we understand much, much more about genetics, biochemistry, inheritance, evolution, and mathematical predictions. The Human Genome Project has sequenced the entire genome of Mendel's garden pea. What we no longer have is a precise understanding of genes and

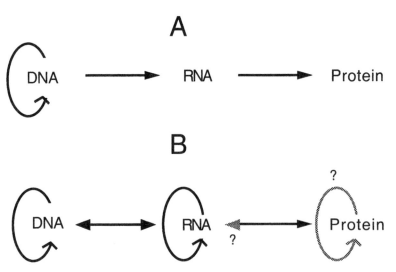

Figure 4.2   The Central Dogma of Biology. A shows the original idea—DNA replicates itself and also defines RNA. The RNA defines the protein. B shows modern thinking—DNA replicates itself and also defines RNA. The RNA can define DNA and protein and can also replicate itself. RNA can also regulate the production and processing of other RNA. Proteins may be able to dictate the structure of RNA and may be able to self-replicate.

how they work. The more we have learned, the more complex the process has become. Now a double strand of DNA is one gene if read in one direction and another if read in the opposite direction. A single gene may be processed into two or more proteins that do significantly different things. It matters whether the gene was inherited from the mother or the father. And the final expression of the gene depends not on the DNA but on the behavior of the RNA or protein toward other RNAs or proteins.

Most simply put today, a gene is a hereditary unit that occupies a specific position within the genome; it has one or more specific effects upon the phenotype (physical features) of an organism; it can mutate into various forms, some of which are benign; and it can combine with other such hereditary units. A gene is a stretch of DNA with its promoters and enhancers that, when transcribed in a particular way, leads to the formation of a particular type of RNA or a protein.

All genes come in pairs. This is not the double strandedness: there are two molecules of identical DNA in each cell. Each of these molecules is a chromosome, which is described in more detail below. So, each gene, each molecule of DNA, has an identical sister gene or molecule in the same cell. The sisters are called alleles (ah-leel). This is true for all higher animals and is thought to have evolved as a backup system and as a way to increase genetic variety and health.

(Geneticists use the terms "gene" and "allele" inconsistently. For this book, "gene" means a stretch of DNA that codes for something and may be present in more than one copy. "Allele" means one of two identical or nearly identical copies of the same gene. The plural of allele is alleles.)

When both alleles of a gene are the same (both normal or both mutated), a person is said to be *homozygous* with respect to that gene. The Greek roots are *homo* = the same and *zygotos* = yoke. So, two of the same thing are joined or yoked together. When one allele has one DNA base sequence and the other has a different one, the person is *heterozygous*: two different things are yoked together. The two heterozygous alleles may be both normal, one normal and one abnormal, or both abnormal.

Homo sapiens is estimated to have 30,000 genes. This is a lot, but not enough to account for the intricate workings of the human body. Each of these genes codes for an RNA or a protein. The RNAs and proteins then work together in a large variety of ways that have almost infinite possible combinations. At the time of this writing, geneticists are only beginning to understand what this really means. Research is moving from the Genome Project to the Proteome Project, which looks at the gene products. It is now thought that the complexity of biologic systems lies not within the DNA but at the level of the DNA products: RNA and protein.

CHROMOSOMES

There is a lot of DNA in each cell of our bodies—roughly six feet. To fit into a cell, that two yards of DNA must be condensed. The DNA is condensed into chromosomes. This condensation is often modeled by using a coiled telephone cord. If such a cord is twisted upon itself it doubles over, forming secondary and tertiary twists. The double helix of DNA is first wrapped around proteins called histones. The histones in human beings are very similar to those in other animals, which suggests that the structure of the histone is very important—it did not change much with evolution. This is called evolutionary conservation of a gene or gene sequence.

The DNA-histone unit is called a nucleosome. The nucleosomes pack into a chromatin fiber that coils and super-coils into the structure we call a chromosome. For most of a cell's lifetime, the chromosomes are not cleanly visible. They are uncoiled in the nucleus of the cell so that the genes can be transcribed and translated and so that DNA itself can be replicated. The chromosomes become more visible during cell division. At that time, they condense as much as possible and are separated into the dividing daughter cells. It is at the time of cell division—mitosis—that chromosomes are most easily seen.

Chromosomes are large molecules of DNA and are visible under a normal microscope. Human beings have twenty-three pairs of chromosomes. Twenty-two pairs are called autosomes. They are the same for everyone and are numbered 1 to 22 from largest to smallest. (Actually, chromosome 21 is the smallest, but by the time that was figured out the numbers were already in place.) The twenty-third pair is the sex chromosomes. Females have two X chromosomes, males have an X chromosome and a Y chromosome. Of each pair, one chromosome is inherited from the mother in the egg and the other comes from the father in the sperm. At fertilization, the maternal and paternal chromosomes form their pairs. Eggs and sperm are the only cells in the body that normally have only half the standard number of chromosomes.

In making gametes, two things happen to all chromosomes that cause us all to be a bit different from each other. The first is that the pairs shuffle. One set of chromosomes is not inherited straight from great grandparent to grandparent to parent to child. From mom, a child may get grandma's chromosome 1, grandpa's chromosome 2, and so forth. Same for the set from dad. The second thing that happens is recombination. At a specific point in the making of egg or sperm, the chromosomes line up side by side and exchange pieces. They literally break, trade, and reseal themselves. This is visible under a microscope as a crossing over of the chromosome arms.

Recombination means that no chromosome is ever inherited exactly the way it was in the parent. The differences are subtle. The result is that there is an infinite possible variety of ways to inherit genes and other genetic material. Recombination has been used as a tool to map genes. There are even small sections at the tip ends of the X and Y chromosomes that are similar enough to cross over and recombine.

Although they are all slightly varied, chromosomes have a standard structure, as shown in Figure 4.3. Chromosomes have a short arm—the p arm—and a long arm—the q arm. (The mnemonic for this is that pints are smaller than quarts.) Between the arms is the centromere, which appears as a waist. In cell division the centromere is the attachment point by which the chromosome is pulled around the cell. Locations on the chromosome arms are labeled relative to their distance from the centromere. Proximal is close to the centromere and distal is farther away. The centromere can be in the middle of the chromosome, off to one side, or very near one end. When the centromere is near one end, as in chromosomes 13, 14, 15, 21, and 22, the p arm is very small.

When the chromosomes are treated with a stain, stripes appear. These stripes are called bands or "G bands" after the stain used. The banding pattern is very stable, so that, in human beings, all chromosomes 1 look alike, all chromosomes 2 look alike, and so on. This is handy for genetic

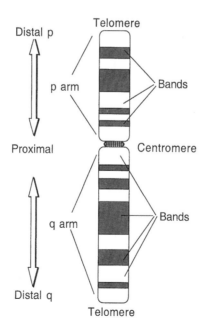

Figure 4.3   Normal chromosome structure.

testing because a patient's chromosomes can be compared against the human species standard. Any extra or missing pieces or rearrangements, therefore, are easier to find. The bands are numbered using a conventional international nomenclature so that precise points along the chromosome may be specified.

The chromosome and band numbers are used as a shorthand. For example, common trisomy 21 in a girl is indicated as 47,XX,+21. Instead of 46 chromosomes there are 47, and the extra one is a 21. A missing piece of the chromosome 8 long arm in a boy can be coded as 46,XY,del(8)(q21).[4] There are also codes for when a piece is duplicated, turned around, stuck somewhere else, and so on. The shorthand system takes practice to master, but it is very precise.

A chromosome analysis, or karyotype, is a common genetic test. It can be performed on any cell that has a nucleus and that divides. The cell has to have a nucleus because that is where the chromosomes are. The cell must be able to grow and divide because that is when the chromosomes are visible. Some cells in the body do not have a nucleus, such as red blood cells. Other cells, such as nerve and muscle cells, do not divide. In the genetics clinic, the karyotype is most often done as a blood test using the white blood cells.

MENDEL WAS ONLY THE BEGINNING

DNA and how it works are much better understood today than even just one hundred years ago. However, the more we learn, the more complex genetic science gets. The basic structures and biochemical interactions are fairly well defined, but the nuances are many. There are multiple levels of increasing complexity: four DNA bases code for twenty amino acids, the amino acids make different proteins when put in different order, and the proteins interact differently depending upon their cellular location, how they are processed, and what other proteins are present. RNA is now found to be more of a stage manager in the cell, regulating proteins, DNA, and other bits of RNA.

Descriptions of inheritance patterns are equally simple and complex. The patterns originally described by Gregor Mendel—the Mendelian inheritance patterns—are still useful today for many conditions. Again, though, there are variations on the themes. Sometimes genetic disease runs in families, which will be discussed in Chapter 6. Other times, genetic disease is hidden, or occurs spontaneously, which is the topic of Chapter 7. Even when a genetic mutation is present, the way it will manifest is not as predictable as we would like.

PART II

Pregnancy and Pregnancy Planning

5 Forewarned and Forearmed

Pregnancy is not a disease. Even with all the emphasis on medicine and hospitals, pregnancy and childbirth are processes that can happen just fine without much medical intervention. Despite that, there are things that can prevent or interfere with normal pregnancy. For many people, their first encounter with genetics outside of school happens because of a pregnancy. There may be questions before conception about a condition that runs in the family or about a health problem in the mother. Infertility or repeated pregnancy losses may prompt a genetics consultation. Prenatal screening or routine ultrasound may suggest a problem that needs further attention.

PLANNED PARENTHOOD

Fifty percent of pregnancies in the United States are unplanned.[1] This is an important point, so it deserves being stated again: in the United States, half of all pregnancies are unplanned. The majority of these are to married couples. All are to women who are not practicing birth control or in whom the birth control has failed. A significant minority are victims of rape, incest, or other abuse.

There are two inherent problems in such a high rate of unplanned pregnancy. The first is that an unplanned pregnancy is more likely to be an unwanted pregnancy. Unwantedness of pregnancy interferes with women seeking prenatal care and results in other ethical and social predicaments that are beyond the scope of this book. The second problem is that an unplanned pregnancy is less likely to start out as a healthy pregnancy. Unplanned pregnancies are at higher risk for preventable conditions.

The embryo is susceptible at any age to genetic and environmental influences. There is an old axiom that the first two weeks after conception is an "all or none" period for the embryo: an exposure either causes miscarriage or does no damage at all. Newer evidence from studies of fetal alcohol exposure has proven this not to be true. Because the very early embryo is the most sensitive, some maternal conditions are best managed or treated even before conception takes place.

An unplanned pregnancy will often not be detected until a month or more after conception. These first twenty-eight days are crucial to the healthy development of the embryo. Maternal deficiency in folic acid contributes to spina bifida, which is established by twenty-eight days and cannot be corrected. Use of alcohol and cigarettes can have a great impact. Most women stop smoking or drinking once they know they are pregnant. But if they do not know they are pregnant until two or three months, much damage may already have been done.

There are two ways to measure the age of a pregnancy. The most common is from the beginning of the mother's last menstrual period—this is the measurement used by obstetricians, other doctors, and the general public. When discussing embryology—the development of the embryo/fetus—the measurement starts at conception. Conception is, on average, two weeks after the last menstrual period. Table 5.1 shows some weeks for comparison.

FERTILITY

First to define some terms. Medically speaking, pregnancy does not begin with conception. Pregnancy is the state in which a fertilized egg (zygote) is successfully implanted in the wall of the uterus. Even in normal, healthy, fertile couples, the odds of starting a pregnancy—having a fertilized egg successfully implant—are only about 30% with each menstrual cycle.

There is a general belief that women of average or better health will have good pregnancies and healthy babies. This is certainly true a lot of the time. If it were not, humans would not survive as a species. More precise measures of fertility show that the natural process is more likely to go wrong than to go right. Fertility problems, miscarriages, infant deaths, and serious birth defects tend to be talked about only within the privacy of the family. In the shopping mall or at the soccer game—the public

Table 5.1 Measuring Pregnancy Age in Two Common But Different Ways

Event	Weeks after LMP[a]	Weeks after conception
Conception	2	0
Implantation in the Uterus (Pregnancy starts)	3	1
Spinal Cord and Brain start to form	4 1/2	2 1/2
Recognizable 4-chamber heart	6 1/2	4 1/2
Chorionic Villus Sampling[b]	10	8
Recognizable face	12	10
Second Trimester	12	10
Early Amniocentesis[b]	13	11
First Ultrasound[b]	16–18	14–16
Regular Amniocentesis[b]	18–20	16–18
Third trimester	24	22
Term delivery	40	38

[a] LMP = Last menstrual period.
[b] These are common tests done during a pregnancy. Not all pregnancies get these tests, and the timing of a test varies from pregnancy to pregnancy. The times stated are most usual.

arenas—the children are usually healthy and whole. This gives the false impression that the ideal is the most common state, when actually it is not. Many things have to go right for pregnancy and development to happen the way we want. Despite appearances, much of the time something goes wrong.

Before the advent of simple urine pregnancy tests, early pregnancy failure was not really recognized. A woman might have a menstrual cycle that was slightly delayed or heavier than usual, but this was seen as a menstrual irregularity. Now it is possible for a woman to confirm a pregnancy as early as one week after implantation—before her expected next period. After that point a late or heavy period is more accurately recognized as an early pregnancy failure.

A majority of zygotes do not implant in the uterine wall and are washed out with the next menstrual cycle. Of those embryos that do implant, as many as half fail in the first few weeks. This equates to about a 50% rate of spontaneous abortion (death or loss of an embryo that has implanted) for all pregnancies. Figure 5.1 provides some rough numbers in the chronology of pregnancy failure or loss. After the first trimester, the chance

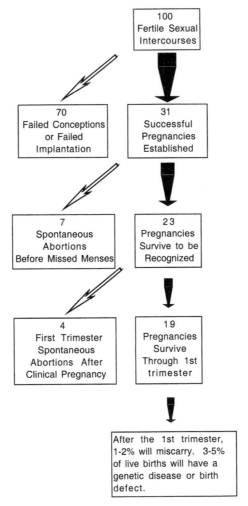

Figure 5.1   Normal fertility.

of spontaneous abortion or stillbirth is 1–2%. The longer the pregnancy continues, the more likely it is to survive to term, but there is never a guarantee. For pregnancies that survive to live birth, there is a 3–5% risk of birth defect or genetic disease identifiable in the first year of life.

The high rate of early pregnancy failure (lack of conception, lack of embryo implantation, or early abortion) is thought to have some genetic basis. Thus, women or couples who have significant infertility or multiple pregnancy losses may be referred for genetic consultation. Abnormal eggs and sperm may not succeed in fertilization. If fertilization happens, the resulting abnormal zygote either does not implant or aborts. It is estimated that half of these losses are due to a genetic abnormality. Thus, the early loss of abnormal embryos is a natural way of selecting for healthy babies.

In some pregnancy losses, it is possible to pinpoint the cause, but for most it is not. Even if a particular genetic abnormality is diagnosed in the fetus, it is not currently possible to say what association there may be between the genetic problem and the fact that the fetus did not survive. In more and more cases, it is possible to predict the chance of the same problem happening in a future pregnancy. The ability to predict complications of the next pregnancy depends upon the ability to diagnose the problem in the current abnormal fetus. The more tests that can be done on an aborted or stillborn fetus—genetic, biochemical, X ray, and autopsy examinations—the more knowledge there can be about the future.

Some environmental agents are known to cause birth defects. The remainder of this chapter will discuss some of these. Avoidance of as many of these agents as possible will increase the chances of a healthy pregnancy and baby.

TERATOGENS

Teratogens (ter-a′-to-jens) are substances—chemicals, infections, radiation, or chronic disease in mom—that cause birth defects. The word comes from the Greek: *terato* (monster) + *gen* (causing/producing). The measure of a substance's ability to cause birth defects is its *teratogenicity*. The study of birth defects caused by such things is *teratology*. Technically, mutated genes are also teratogens, but in common usage "teratogen" means something to which the fetus is exposed rather than a genetic mutation.

As stated above, one well-established way to have a healthy pregnancy is to prepare for it. A frequently used analogy points out that people generally put more time, research, and effort into buying a new car than in preparing for a pregnancy. For the benefit of the child, planning for that child should begin before conception rather than after the positive pregnancy test. The first two months of pregnancy are even more important than a good day care center or the right car seat.

Timing of a pregnancy allows the mother's body to be as healthy as possible to support the pregnancy. Controlling a chronic health problem, or just recovering physically and nutritionally from a previous pregnancy, can go a long way. Typically, it is recommended that the mother be ready to support a pregnancy a minimum of three months prior to conception. That means, three months before having intercourse with the intent of becoming pregnant, the mother should be taking care of herself as well as if she were already pregnant.

This recommendation arose from the care of diabetic women: strict control of diabetes at least three months prior to conception appeared to decrease (but not eliminate) risks to both the mother and the fetus. This paradigm has been translated into all other situations: three months off of birth control pills, three months of good vitamin intake, and so on. There is no scientific support for this specific time span in every instance; it may be too short a time for some things and overkill for others. But three months is a useful length because it is easy to remember—it is a season, or one-quarter of a year, or equivalent to one trimester of pregnancy.

The degree to which a teratogen causes problems depends upon the following:

1. Duration of exposure—how long the embryo/fetus is exposed.
2. Level of exposure—how much of the substance is present at a given time.
3. Timing of exposure—when during the pregnancy the exposure took place.
4. Sensitivity of the fetus—genetic makeup and metabolism of the fetus.
5. Metabolism of the mother—how well the mother's body can protect the fetus.
6. Mechanism of teratogenicity—biochemically, how the agent causes a problem.

Items 4, 5, and 6 are unmeasurable. Because of this, it is impossible to say whether exposure to a teratogen will definitely cause a particular defect. Some fetuses will be exposed quite a bit without much or any problem. Other fetuses with only minimal or transient exposure will have severe effects. Some things are absolutes: thalidomide taken during the first trimester will cause limb abnormalities, alcohol taken in significant quantity at any time will cause mental retardation. More detailed diagnoses have to wait until the fetus or infant can be examined. Table 5.2 lists some known teratogens and the problems that they cause.

Some infections are teratogenic. It should be noted that these are infections, not vaccinations. Vaccinations are not routinely given to pregnant women because all vaccines carry the risk that they might cause an infection. The vaccinations themselves, working as they are supposed to, are not a risk. Sometimes the risk of getting a disease is very high—for example, if there is an active rubella or smallpox outbreak in the community. In that circumstance, the risk of disease is higher than the risk of vaccine side effect, so pregnant women will be offered the vaccine.

More often, the risk of getting the disease is low, so vaccinations are not given to pregnant women. Rubella infection (German measles) while pregnant causes the problems indicated in Table 5.2. It is a routine part of prenatal care to test whether the pregnant woman is immune to rubella. Most women are immune because they received the vaccination as a child. If a woman is not immune, and there is not an outbreak in the community, she will be vaccinated after she delivers the baby. In this

Table 5.2   Teratogens: External Agents That Cause Birth Defects

	Teratogen	Birth Defects
I N F E C T I O N S	Cytomegalovirus (CMV)	Small head, blindness, mental retardation, fetal death
	Herpes	Small eyes, small head, abnormal retina
	Rubella (German measles)	Cataracts, glaucoma, heart defects, deafness
	Syphilis	Mental retardation, deafness, bone abnormalities
	Toxoplasmosis	Hydrocephalus, brain calcifications, small eyes
	Varicella (chicken pox)	Limb growth abnormalities, mental retardation, skin abnormalities
	Variola major (smallpox)	Unknown, presumed to be a teratogen
	Variola minor (cowpox)	Possible limb abnormalities and small head
M I S C	X-rays/radiation	Small head, spina bifida, cleft palate, limb defects
	Hyperthermia	Anencephaly (missing brain)
C H E M I C A L S	ACE inhibitors (Heart drugs)	Growth retardation, fetal death
	Alcohol	"Fetal alcohol syndrome" abnormal face, heart defects, mental retardation
	Aminopterin (Cancer drug)	Anencephaly, hydrocephaly, cleft lip and palate
	Amphethamines	Cleft lip and palate, heart defects
	Androgenic agents	Masculinization of female genitalia
	Cocaine	Growth retardation, small head, abnormal behavior, opening in the abdominal wall (gastroschsis)
	Diethylstilbestrol (DES)	Malformation of female genitalia, vaginal cancer, malformed testes
	Diphenylhydantoin (Dilantin)	"Fetal hydantoin syndrome" facial abnormalities, mental retardation, missing nails/short digits
	Isotretinoin (Retinoic acid)	Small abnormal ears, small jaw, cleft palate, heart defects.
	Lead	Growth retardation, neurologic disorders
	Lithium (Anti-psychotic)	Heart defects
	Mercury	Neurologic defects
	Thalidomide (Leprosy drug)	Limb defects, heart defects
	Trimethadone (Cancer drug)	Cleft palate, heart defects, defects of the skeleton, genitalia, and urinary system
	Valproic Acid (Seizure drug)	Spina bifida, heart and limb defects, facial abnormalities
	Warfarin (Anti-clotting drug)	Abnormal cartilage, small head

Note: All defects do not happen in all exposed fetuses. Please refer to the text for factors that contribute to teratogenicity.

instance, the risk of getting the disease is roughly zero and the risk of a vaccine complication is above zero, even though it is very small.

Many teratogens are avoidable but are used anyway. The best study done to date notes that almost half of women drink alcohol in the first three months of their pregnancy because they do not yet know that they are pregnant.[2] Alcohol's effects on the fetus are well documented in many studies, and there is no known safe minimum amount. Even when there are no physical defects, prenatal alcohol exposure can cause IQ deficit and behavior problems. Smoking is recognized to cause growth retardation in the fetus, increase the risk of many pregnancy complications, including premature birth[3] and sudden infant death syndrome, and may be linked to autism.[4] Cigarette smoking also increases the risk of birth defects such as cleft lip.

Illicit drugs are more difficult to study because they are rarely taken alone. Most women who use cocaine, for example, also use tobacco and/or alcohol. Cocaine is known to be associated with nervous system and behavioral problems. When used heavily or in early pregnancy, it is associated with some physical defects such as missing digits or other problems. It has been suggested that cocaine causes constriction of blood vessels in the fetus. If the blood supply to an organ or body part is compromised, it fails to develop correctly.

Sometimes the teratogen is not avoidable. For example, if the mother has seizures, it is important for her to be on medication. Some seizure medications are teratogens. To minimize the risk of teratogenicity, she may be put on another medication or the blood levels of her medication may be closely monitored. In all cases, the risk to the mother and the risk to the fetus must be balanced. While it is not good to expose the fetus to a teratogen, it is worse to leave the mother open to having seizures. A pregnant woman diagnosed with cancer faces a similar dilemma.

Sometimes, a woman will have a chronic disease that can be a teratogen. Table 5.3 lists some of these diseases. These diseases are not avoidable but should be controlled as much as possible before and during a pregnancy. The risks to the fetus are in addition to whatever risk pregnancy itself might cause to the mother. Sometimes the risk to the fetus may be minimal but pregnancy is dangerous to the mother or may worsen the mother's disease.

MINIMIZING RISK

Even for healthy, fertile couples, the chance in any month of a successful pregnancy and healthy baby are low. Many reasons that pregnancies

Table 5.3   Teratogens: Chronic Disease in the Mother

Disease	Birth Defects
Juvenile (Type 1) Diabetes	'Mermaid' syndrome - abnormal formation of lower half of body
Adult (Type 2) Diabetes	Overgrowth of baby
Folic acid deficiency	Neural Tube defects - spina bifida and anencephaly
Hyperthyroidism	**Thought to increase overall risk**
Hypothyroidism	**Thought to increase overall risk**
Immune-mediated thrombocytopenia	Low platelet count and bleeding problems
Myesthenia Gravis	Neonatal myesthenia
Phenylketonuria (PKU)	Small head, mental retardation
Sjögren syndrome	Conduction defects of the heart, abnormal heart beat
Systemic Lupus Erythematosis (SLE)	Conduction defects of the heart, abnormal heart beat
Virilizing tumors	Masculinization of female fetus

fail are known or surmised to be genetic. Of those pregnancies that are successful, half are unplanned, which makes them all the more susceptible to early detrimental exposures or malnutrition. Prepregnancy and periconceptional planning can increase the chance of a healthy fetus because the mother can control any chronic diseases, avoid alcohol, and begin appropriate vitamin supplementation.

There is actually very little known about why conceptions fail or why so many zygotes and embryos abort early in pregnancy. For political reasons, research on human zygotes and embryos and early human pregnancies are not allowed in the United States. Without the answers that such research would generate, there will continue to be limited knowledge about pregnancy failure and fetal loss.

6 When Genetic Disease Runs in a Family

In Chapter 3 there was a short discussion of multifactorial conditions—maladies that arise because of both genetic and environmental influences. These can recur in families but do not follow any particular pattern. Here we will look at some other ways that genetic conditions can affect more than one member of a family. Most of the chapter will discuss the common Mendelian inheritance patterns. Some chromosome problems can be inherited. And there are two special situations—sex-linked inheritance and mitochondrial inheritance.

FAMILY HISTORY OF A DOMINANT CONDITION

When a dominant condition runs in a family, it appears in more than one generation. It can appear that the disease "skips" a generation for reasons outlined in Appendix B. Sometimes parents and grandparents are mildly affected, so they do not know that they have the diagnosis. In these cases, features of the condition may be thought of just as family traits: lots of people in the family are short, or have funny ears, or get these little skin spots. Figure 6.1 shows a typical dominant inheritance family pedigree.

In families like these, there is often no suspicion of a potential problem because no one is really abnormal. It is not unusual for the rest of the family to be diagnosed only when a child is born with a severe form of the condition. That child is referred to a geneticist or other specialty doctor who makes the diagnosis (because it is very obvious in the severe

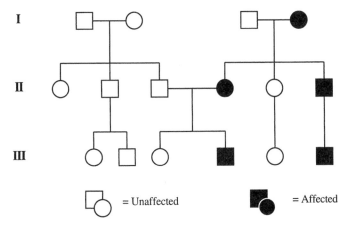

Figure 6.1 Typical pedigree of dominant inheritance. Affected persons are all blood-related. Note that the disease appears in more than one generation and in persons of both sexes. Transmission from father to son is a clue for dominant inheritance rather than X-linked inheritance (see Figure 6.7 for comparison). Note that not all offspring of an affected person are themselves affected. Spouses were not all drawn in the interest of space. Please refer to Figure 2.2 for an explanation of the symbols.

case). The doctor can then review the family history and conclude that others have the same thing. This can come as something of a shock to people who had no idea that they have a genetic disease. Suddenly knowing about a familial gene mutation does not change who the person is, but it does give information. This knowledge may answer questions about chronic health problems. It will also help people make informed decisions about having children.

A dominant disease happens because a gene mutation was present at or soon after conception. This is true even if the disease symptoms do not show up until adulthood. An embryo can come to have a dominant mutation in one of two ways: inheritance from a parent, or a new mutation in the egg or sperm. Here we will discuss inheritance of a dominant disease from a parent. New mutations are discussed in Chapter 7.

DOMINANT INHERITANCE

Figure 6.2 shows the way that a dominant gene mutation can pass from parent to child. Genes come in pairs. The individual copies are alleles, so each person has two alleles for each gene. In a dominant disease, only one allele of the pair needs to be mutated for the disease to show itself. Another way to say this is that persons affected with domi-

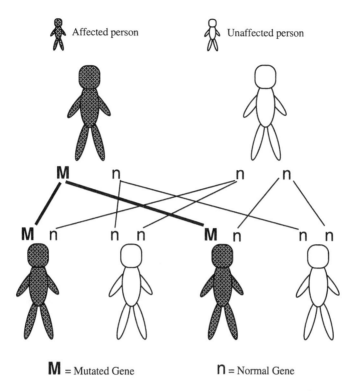

M = Mutated Gene   n = Normal Gene

Figure 6.2   Dominant inheritance, one parent affected (see text for explanation).

nant diseases are heterozygotes—they have one normal and one mutated allele. The one normal allele is insufficient to make up for the mutated allele—this is called a "loss-of-function" mutation. Disease arises because of the lost function of one allele. Sometimes, the mutated allele actively interferes with the workings of the normal one—this is a "dominant negative" mutation.

In the figure, the normal allele is represented by a lowercase "n" and the mutant allele is represented by a capital "M." Capitalization indicates that the mutant allele is dominant over the normal allele. (Please note that "m" and "n" will be used again later in discussions of recessive disease, but in that case the capitalization will be reversed and the normal allele will be dominant over the mutant one.)

When one parent has a dominant condition, that parent is a heterozygote (has one normal allele and one mutated allele). Either allele may be passed to a child. If the normal allele is passed on, the child does not inherit the condition. If the mutated allele is passed on, then the child is affected by the same thing as the parent. The chance of passing on one allele or the other is 50:50 in each pregnancy—the same as a coin toss. On average, half of the children will be affected and half will be unaffected. It is the same risk for both boys and girls.

In the Figure 6.2 example, one parent has the mutation and the other is normal. In Figure 6.3, both parents are affected and have a mutated allele for the same gene. There is still a 1/2, 50:50, or 50% chance that a child will be heterozygous like the parents, but now there is only a 1/4 or 25% chance that the child will be homozygous normal. When both parents have a mutated allele, there is a 1/4 or 25% chance that a child will inherit both mutations—that is, be homozygous for the mutation. In many cases, this means that the child will be more severely affected and the condition may not be survivable. Achondroplasia is like this.

Dominant genetic conditions include achondroplasia (a type of dwarfism), neurofibromatosis (a disease of small skin tumors, pigmented spots, and sometimes brain tumors), Marfan syndrome (tall stature, dislocated eye lenses, and blood vessel abnormalities), and polycystic kidney disease

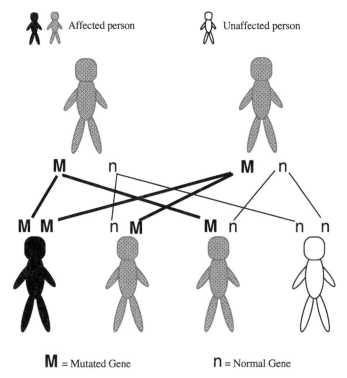

Figure 6.3 Dominant inheritance, both parents affected (see text for explanation).

Table 6.1   Some Dominant Diseases, Their Features, and Their Genes

Disease	Features	Gene
Achondroplasia (Ach[a])	Short limbed dwarfism	Fibroblast Growth Factor Receptor 3
Acrocephalosyndactyly I (Apert)	Early fusion of skull bones, abnormal digits	Fibroblast Growth Factor Receptor 2 (FGFR2)
Familial Hypercholesterolemia with Hyperlipidemia	High blood cholesterol, Extreme risk of heart attack	Apolipoprotein E (ApoE)
Mandibulofacial Dysostosis (Treacher Collins syndrome, TCS)	Missing cheekbones, abnormal eyelids, cleft palate	Treacle (TCOF1)
Marfan syndrome	Tall, loose joints, dislocated lenses, heart/artery problems	Fibrillin
Myotonic Dystrophy 1 (Dystrophia Myotonica, DM1)	Difficulty relaxing muscles, cataracts, abnormal heart/gonads	Dystrophia Myotonica Protein Kinase (DMPK)
Neurofibromatosis, type 1 (NF1)	Spots and tumors on the skin, problems in nerves, bone, muscle	Neurofibromin
Polycystic Kidney Disease - Autosomal Dominant (ADPKD)	Multiple cysts in both kidneys, renal failure, abnormal blood vessels in the brain	There are two genes: Polycystin 1 Polycystin 2
Tuberous Sclerosis (TSC)	Spots and tumors on skin, brain tumors, abnormal kidneys	Multiple genes can cause this: TSC1, TSC2, TSC3 and TSC4
Waardenburg syndrome 1 (WS1)	Pigment abnormalities, deafness, characteristic face	PAX3

[a] The letters in parentheses are common abbreviations or nicknames for these diseases and their genes.

(the most common genetic cause of renal failure). These and other dominant genetic diseases with their identified genes are listed in Table 6.1. There are hundreds of dominant conditions, so Table 6.1 has examples only.

FAMILY HISTORY OF A RECESSIVE CONDITION

When a recessive genetic condition runs in a family, it usually appears in siblings. Rather than being in multiple generations, it is all in one generation. It can be present in other people, like grandparents or cousins, but it almost never moves from parent to child. Figure 6.4 shows how a recessive disease appears in a family pedigree.

Recurrent recessive disease in children is most apparent when their parents are consanguineous—are blood relatives to each other. This blood relationship is only rarely incest or other social deviance. Most commonly, consanguinity happens in closed religious communities (such as the Amish, Hasidic Jewish enclaves), small socially isolated communities (such as Cajuns), or when marriages are arranged for the purpose of controlling property inheritance (such as historic Middle Eastern practices). In these communities, there are often well-established rules about

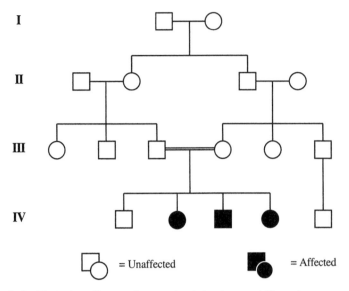

I

II

III

IV

= Unaffected   = Affected

Figure 6.4 Typical pedigree of recessive inheritance. Affected persons are all blood-related. Note that the disease appears in only one generation, but in persons of both sexes. There is consanguinity—the parents of the affected children are first cousins. Recessive disease is more likely when there is consanguinity, but it can appear in any family. Please refer to Figure 2.2 for an explanation of the symbols.

who may mate with whom, but the rules do not eliminate the risk of having children affected with recessive disease.[1]

A recessive condition happens because the mutation was present on both alleles of the gene before conception. Speaking very broadly, recessive conditions tend to be more severe than dominant ones, although this is not a clear distinction. Recessive conditions are more commonly diagnosed in infancy or childhood. Although new mutations can happen, the vast majority of recessive disease is inherited from the parents.

RECESSIVE INHERITANCE

When a child is diagnosed with a recessive condition, each of the parents is, by definition, a carrier of a mutated allele for that gene. While there can be a new mutation, it is rare. Making the assumption that both parents are carriers will be correct the vast majority of the time. Figure 6.5 shows how a recessive mutation is inherited. In this example, the "m" (for "mutation") is a lowercase letter because it is recessive to the "N" ("normal") allele.

Both parents are heterozygotes—they both have one normal allele and one mutant allele. When the disease is recessive, the one normal allele is sufficient for normal cell and body function. People who are heterozygous for a recessive disease usually do not know it because they have no symptoms. However, if both parents pass the same mutated gene to their child, that child is affected with the condition.

Once it is known that there is a recessive disease in the family, the risk to each subsequent pregnancy is 1/4 or 25%. This is the chance that the fetus will inherit both mutations and be affected with the condition as its older sibling is. There is a 1/4 or 25% chance that the fetus will inherit both normal alleles. And there is a 2/4 or 1/2 or 50% chance that the fetus will inherit one mutant and one normal allele and be a heterozygous carrier like the parent. These risks are the same for each pregnancy. Having had one affected (or normal) child does not change the risk to the next child. Each pregnancy must be thought of as a new coin toss or dice roll.

If one parent is affected and the other is homozygous normal, then all of the children will be heterozygous carriers. None of them will be

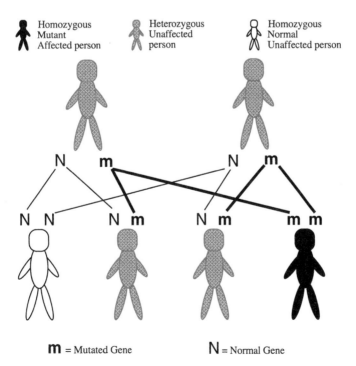

Figure 6.5   Recessive inheritance, neither parent affected (see text for explanation).

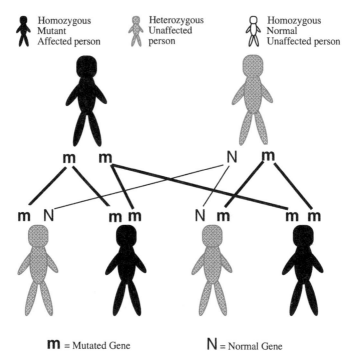

Homozygous Mutant Affected person

Heterozygous Unaffected person

Homozygous Normal Unaffected person

m = Mutated Gene   N = Normal Gene

Figure 6.6   Recessive inheritance, one parent affected (see text for explanation).

clinically affected. When the children grow up, it will be important for them to know that they carry this mutated allele so they will have information for their own family planning.

When one parent is affected with a recessive condition, as in Figure 6.6, and the other parent is a carrier, the risk to the fetus increases. The affected parent can only pass on the mutated gene—there is not a normal version of the gene in this parent. The carrier parent can pass on either the normal or the mutant gene. There is a 1/2 or 50% chance for each pregnancy that a fetus will be affected—that is, homozygous for the mutation. There is a 1/2 or 50% chance for each pregnancy that the fetus will be a heterozygous carrier. When one parent is affected and the other is a carrier, there is no chance that the offspring will be homozygous normal.

CHROMOSOME PROBLEMS

Abnormalities in chromosomes are really large abnormalities in DNA. Problems can involve whole chromosomes, large or small parts of a chromosome, or more than one chromosome. Table 6.2 defines some

Table 6.2   Common Terms Used to Describe Chromosome Problems

Aneuploidy: Any variation from the normal total number of forty-six chromosomes.

Deletion: A missing chromosome or piece of a chromosome.

Duplication: An extra chromosome or piece of a chromosome.

Euploidy: Having the normal number of chromosomes—forty-six in human beings.

Haploidy: Having only one set of chromosomes. Having a total of twenty-three chromosomes rather than forty-six. This is not compatible with life except that normal gametes (eggs and sperm) are haploid.

Inversion: A piece of chromosome that has been cut out, turned around, and reinserted into place.

Monosomy: Missing one of a pair of chromosomes. Having one copy of a given chromosome instead of the normal two. If only part of the chromosome is missing, this is called a "partial monosomy."

Translocation: A chromosome or piece of chromosome that has been moved from its normal location and attached to another chromosome.

Triploidy: An entire extra set of chromosomes. Having a total of sixty-nine chromosomes rather than forty-six.

Trisomy: Having an extra single chromosome. Having three copies of a given chromosome instead of just two. If only part of a chromosome is extra, this is called a "partial trisomy."

common terms used to describe chromosome problems. Some chromo-some problems can affect more than one family member. Sometimes this happens by chance. Trisomy 21 (Down syndrome) is very common—about 1 in every 660 live births. So, it is possible that an extended family could have two children with trisomy 21 simply by chance.

Uncommonly, chromosome problems can be inherited, so they can occur in more than one family member, usually siblings. It is important to know that recurrent chromosome problems are the exception rather than the rule. Most chromosome problems do not run in families. The discussion here is for the minority of cases.

Chromosome problems recur in families because of a translocation. In translocations, large sections of chromosomes are rearranged. Some translocations can involve an entire chromosome. Translocations can be balanced or unbalanced. A balanced translocation is a rearrangement of the genetic material without any gain or loss of DNA. The chromosomes are not in their normal arrangement, but the cell still has the right amount of genetic material. In an unbalanced translocation there is a gain or loss of DNA, so the cell has an abnormal amount of genetic material. Usually, unbalanced translocations result in birth defect, stillbirth, or spontaneous abortion.

When someone has a balanced translocation, he or she is normal. The right amount of DNA and, overall, the right number of chromosomes are present. As such, the cell has all it needs to function, so the balanced translocation carrier usually does not know that this rearrangement exists. The problem arises in the making of the gametes—the eggs or the sperm.

Gametes are formed by a specialized type of cell division called meiosis (my-oh-sis). In the process of meiosis, the chromosome pairs are split apart so that each gamete ends up with only one sister of each pair. Each gamete has 23 chromosomes—one of each number. When the male and female gametes (sperm and egg) fuse at conception, the zygote then has the right number of chromosomes—46 or two of each number.

During meiosis, the cell must be able to recognize each chromosome so that the appropriate division can take place. When there is a translocation, two different chromosomes are stuck together and the cell machinery gets confused. For example, say a large piece of chromosome 1 and a large piece of chromosome 18 have changed places. This is called a reciprocal translocation. As long as this translocation is balanced, there are no problems. When meiosis happens, the cell may treat the translocated chromosome incorrectly—it will not pair up and divide off as it should. As a result, the gamete and ultimately the zygote ends up with an unbalanced translocation.

There are 4 possible ways that a reciprocally translocated chromosome can be treated in meiosis, so there are 4 possible outcomes after fertilization (Figure 6.7). There is 1 chance in 4 that the zygote (fetus) will get all the normal chromosomes and be normal. There is 1 chance in 4 that the zygote will get the translocation in a balanced fashion and be like the parent. Then there are 2 chances in 4 (or 1/2 chance) that the zygote will get an unbalanced translocation and be abnormal. With a few exceptions, zygotes and fetuses with unbalanced translocations do not survive and will spontaneously abort or be stillborn.

There is a special type of translocation called Robertsonian translocation in which two entire chromosomes are stuck together (Figure 6.8). Again, this can be balanced or unbalanced. With Robertsonian translocations, there is a greater risk to the fetus. After fertilization there is 1 chance in 6 that the fetus will be normal. There is 1 chance in 6 that the fetus will be a balanced translocation carrier like the parent. Then there

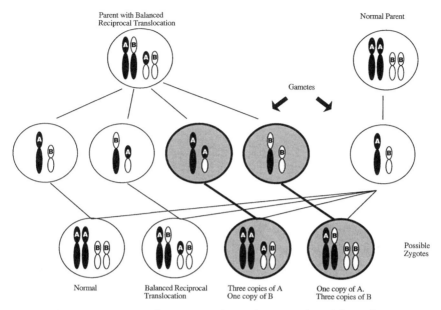

Figure 6.7 Inheritance of a reciprocal translocation. A and B can be any two chromosomes. To simplify the figure, only the chromosomes involved in the translocation are shown. All other chromosomes should be considered normal. The unbalanced gametes and zygotes are indicated by heavy lines and gray background. The parent with the balanced translocation can make four kinds of gametes—one kind with each of the four possible chromosome combinations. One is normal, one is balanced, and two are unbalanced. The normal parent makes only one kind of gamete. (The normal parent does not make fewer gametes, just fewer types of gametes.) When the gametes fuse at conception, there are four possible outcomes: normal (two copies of each chromosome in normal arrangement), balanced translocation, trisomy (three copies) of A/monosomy (one copy) of B, and monosomy A/trisomy B.

are 4 chances in 6 (or 2/3 chance) that the fetus will get an unbalanced translocation and be abnormal. Robertsonian translocations always involve the acrocentric chromosomes (chromosomes with the centromeres at one end) 13, 14, 15, 21, and 22.

The most common Robertsonian translocation in live-born children involves chromosomes 14 and 21. When the translocation is unbalanced and results in three copies of chromosome 21, then the baby has Down syndrome. About 10% of children who have Down syndrome have a translocation. The extra chromosome 21 is most often translocated onto a 14 or a 13, or two 21 chromosomes are stuck together. Rarely, the extra chromosome 21 will be translocated onto another one of the chromosomes, but that will not be a regular translocation, not a Robertsonian one.

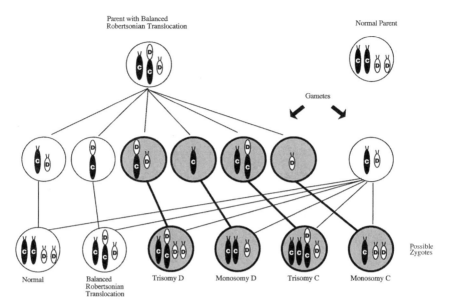

Figure 6.8 Inheritance of a Robertsonian translocation. C and D can be any two acrocentric chromosomes—chromosomes with their centromeres at the ends. The acrocentric chromosomes are 13, 14, 15, 21, and 22. To simplify the figure, only the chromosomes involved in the translocation are shown. All other chromosomes should be considered normal. The unbalanced gametes and zygotes are indicated by heavy lines and gray background. The parent with the balanced translocation can make six kinds of gametes—one kind with each of the six possible chromosome combinations. One is normal, one is balanced, and four are unbalanced. The normal parent makes only one kind of gamete. (The normal parent does not make fewer gametes, just fewer types of gametes.) When the gametes fuse at conception, there are six possible outcomes: normal (two copies of each chromosome in normal arrangement), balanced translocation (two copies of each chromosome in translocation), trisomy (three copies) of D, monosomy (one copy) of D, trisomy C, and monosomy C.

Most fetuses that have unbalanced translocations spontaneously abort. When a parent has a balanced translocation, one sign is that the mother has multiple miscarriages. This is why women who have had two or more pregnancy losses might be referred for genetic evaluation.

The most common genetic cause of pregnancy loss is thought to be trisomy 16—an embryo with three copies of chromosome 16. This causes severe early disruption of the embryo and never allows development past a few days after conception. Monosomy X—having just one sex chromosome, frequently called Turner syndrome—is another common cause of spontaneous abortion.

SEX-LINKED CONDITIONS

Until now, this chapter has dealt with genes on the autosomes—the chromosomes that are the same in both males and females. There are also genes on the sex chromosomes—the X and the Y. These genes are called "sex-linked" because their effects are determined by whether a person is male or female. The inheritance patterns of these genes will be discussed in more detail in Chapter 13.

When a sex-linked condition runs in a family, it is usually on the X chromosome and mostly shows up in males. Females, having two X chromosomes, tend to be carriers—they have one mutated allele and one normal allele for the X-linked gene. Most genes on the X chromosome do not have partners on the Y. When a male inherits a mutated allele on his X chromosome, there is no normal allele to take up the slack. The male is said to be *hemizygous* for the gene or mutation.

When X-linked conditions run in a family, they are never passed from father to son. The father passes only his Y chromosome to his son, never his X. (Using the family pedigree, this is a handy way to tell an X-linked condition from a dominant one.) Usually the disease shows up in two of a woman's male relatives—such as her brother and her son—while she is unaffected. Figure 6.9 shows a typical pattern of sex-linked inheritance for genes on the X chromosome. Figure 6.10 shows sex-linked inheritance for genes on the Y chromosome. Notice that, in the latter, no females are affected (females do not inherit a Y chromosome) and that the condition passes from a father to all of his sons.

MITOCHONDRIAL CONDITIONS

There is also a set of diseases caused by abnormalities in a special type of DNA. Within the cell is an organelle (small organ of the cell) called a mitochondrion (plural, mitochondria). Mitochondria produce the energy molecules that drive various cell functions, so they are called the "power houses" of the cell. Mitochondria evolved from bacteria that came to live inside animal cells and they still have their own DNA. Mitochondrial DNA (mtDNA) is similar to the DNA of bacteria—it is double stranded and circular. When there is a mutation in the mtDNA, it usually interferes with the cell's ability to produce energy and do its work. Diseases caused by mtDNA mutations affect organs and tissues with high energy requirements, such as the heart, brain, muscle, and eye.

Mitochondria reproduce on their own within cells. They are not dependent upon cellular division. The number of mitochondria in a cell depends upon the function of that cell. Body tissues with high energy

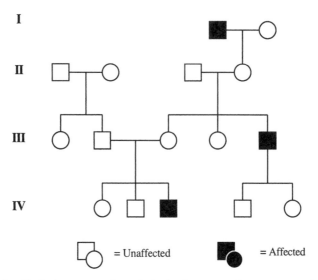

Figure 6.9 Typical pattern of sex-linked inheritance for genes on the X chromosome. Affected persons are all blood-related. Note that the disease appears in more than one generation, but only in males. There is no transmission of the disease from father to son. The females between affected males must be carriers of the mutation. Spouses were not all drawn in the interest of space. Please refer to Figure 2.2 for an explanation of the symbols.

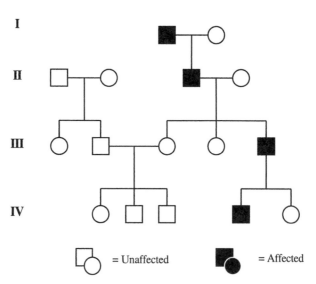

Figure 6.10 Typical pattern of sex-linked inheritance for genes on the Y chromosome. Affected persons are all blood-related. Note that the disease appears in more than one generation, but only in males. There is only transmission of the disease from father to son. Spouses were not all drawn in the interest of space. Please refer to Figure 2.2 for an explanation of the symbols.

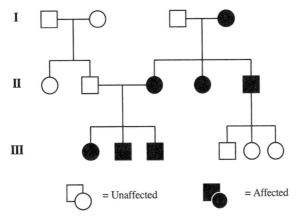

Figure 6.11 Typical pattern of mitochondrial inheritance. Affected persons are all blood-related. Note that the disease appears in more than one generation, in persons of both sexes. There is only transmission of the disease from affected women, and then all of their children are affected. Affected men do not pass on the condition. Spouses were not all drawn in the interest of space. Please refer to Figure 2.2 for an explanation of the symbols.

needs—such as heart muscle—have hundreds, maybe thousands, of mitochondria in each cell. Other tissues with low energy needs—such as hair follicles—have tens or dozens of mitochondria.

All of a person's mitochondria are inherited from the mother in the egg. The egg has dozens to hundreds of mitochondria that become part of the next generation. Sperm do not contribute any mitochondria to a zygote. When a mitochondrial mutation runs in a family, it appears only in children of affected women. Affected men do not pass on the condition to children of either sex (this is different from sex-linked disease)—it stops with them. Figure 6.11 shows a typical pattern for mitochondrial inheritance. This is also called a "maternal inheritance" pattern because affected children get the disease only from their mothers.

Mitochondrial mutations can be difficult to diagnose. It is even more difficult to know what the recurrence risk is (the chance that the next fetus/child will be affected) or how severe the case may be in a given individual. There are two specific reasons that predication is difficult:

1. In each cell there are many mitochondria. Not all mitochondria will have a mutation. If a cell has just a few affected mitochondria, the cell may not be abnormal at all. If many cells in a tissue are like this, then the tissue will not be affected. On the other hand, if a cell has many mutated mitochondria, it will not be able to function normally,

and many such cells will impair tissue function. Unfortunately, it is impossible to predict the distribution of affected mitochondria in a cell or affected cells in a tissue.

2. In each mitochondrion, there are many copies of mtDNA. In a given mitochondrion, all, some, or none of the mtDNA copies may be mutated. Again, severity of disease is dependent upon how many mutated copies are present. Unfortunately, this is impossible to predict.

Mitochondrial conditions are possibly more numerous than currently thought. The symptoms can be sporadic and overlap with other, more common conditions, such as infections and toxic exposure. There are some blood biochemical abnormalities, but these are not unique to mitochondrial problems. Diagnosis is best made when there is a high index of suspicion and direct testing of mitochondrial function or mtDNA sequence.

THINKING OF PATTERNS

Many genetic diseases have specific inheritance patterns. When a pattern can be established, it increases the chance that the correct diagnosis can be made. It also allows for better recurrence prediction. Sometimes it can be surprising to find that there is something running in the family. A set of problems or physical features can be present in a family for generations without being considered unusual. At some point, a much more severely affected child is born. Evaluation of the parents and grandparents shows that, in fact, the condition has been present for a long time.

7 Hidden Genetic Risks

Genetic disease can appear in a new baby even though no one else in the family is affected. For many conditions and many families, this is the rule rather than the exception. Chapter 6 discussed the situations in which genetic disease can run in the family. This chapter will look at the ways that a disease can seem suddenly to appear. There are two basic ways—a new mutation in the genetic material, or confluence of previously "hidden" mutations.

NEW MUTATION IN DOMINANT DISEASE

Changes in the genetic material—mutations—happen continuously. Most of these changes are repaired by the cell, or they occur in a place that does not matter. A very small number of the changes can be traced back to some exposure, such as to radiation or chemicals. For the vast majority of mutations, the cause is unknown.

In dominant conditions, new mutation causes disease. There is not any history of the condition in the family because the mutation did not exist in the family before. There is no way to predict that a particular mutation will happen. There is no way to prevent a mutation from happening. Mutations most often happen in the egg or the sperm. Thus, the change is present before conception ever takes place.

Sometimes a mutation happens soon after conception. This is called a *somatic mutation*. It may or may not involve the gonads, so it may or may not be heritable. Somatic mutation may cause an isolated birth defect or a syndrome. Somatic mutations can play a part in the expressivity of a condition (see Appendix B).

Dominant conditions caused by new mutations are more likely to happen when fathers are older. This is the "paternal age effect." Older fathers, particularly those over forty, are at increased risk for having sperm with a mutation. Advanced paternal age, empirically about thirty-seven and a half years, has been associated with achondroplasia, Apert syndrome, schizophrenia, and some congenital heart diseases.

If a new dominant mutation happens in one child, the mutation is limited to the affected child. The parents are not at risk of having another child with the same problem. However, when the affected child grows up, his or her risk of having offspring with the same condition is 50% (see Figure 6.2). We often think of some condition in a family starting with "Great Grandpa Joe." It is hard to think about future inherited problems as starting with an infant or child. Someday, though, that baby may be a grandparent who is identified as the first person in the family with the genetic mutation.

As with many things, there is an exception to the rule here. Sometimes a new dominant disease can happen in more than one child in the family even though the parents are genetically normal. This phenomenon is known as *gonadal mosaicism*. Briefly, this means that the parent's body cells are genetically normal, but the cells that make the eggs or sperm have a mutation. The parent is not affected with the condition but is at significant risk to have affected children. Unfortunately, there is no easy way to test for gonadal mosaicism, and it is usually only discovered after the birth of a second affected child. Fortunately, it is rare.

NEW RECESSIVE

Recessive diseases usually do not run in families, unless the family is small and has many generations of cousins marrying cousins. Unlike dominant diseases, new recessive diseases are not caused by new mutations in the DNA. When a newborn is diagnosed with a recessive disease, the assumption is made that both parents are carriers of the condition.

We all carry 8 or 10 or 14 gene mutations that are potentially detrimental. Since these mutations are recessive, and genes come in allele pairs, the normal sister allele makes up the difference. As a result, we can have these mutations and not know it—our bodies are normal. The problem arises when we happen to have children with someone who carries one of the same mutations that we do. Then, unbeknownst to the parents, there is a 25% risk with each pregnancy that the fetus will inherit both mutations and be affected with a recessive disease.

Because these mutations are hidden, there is no way of anticipating the birth of an affected child. We do not control what genes we pass to children. There is no way to predict precisely that a child will inherit a mutation or a normal gene. There is no way to prevent it from happening when it happens. Most recessive diseases are very, very rare, and the chance of two parents randomly carrying the same mutation is extremely low. It should be remembered, though, that no risk is zero.

Some recessive diseases are relatively common: sickle cell in persons of African descent, cystic fibrosis in those from northern Europe, Tay-Sachs disease in Ashkenazi Jews and Cajuns. There are tests available to determine whether someone is a carrier for these mutations. Carrier screening is more and more commonly offered to couples having or considering a pregnancy. The screening is tailored to the couple's ethnic group because those are the persons most at risk. For example, the standard "Jewish screen"[1] is for cystic fibrosis, Tay-Sachs disease, Gaucher disease, and Canavan disease.

CHROMOSOMES

Sporadic chromosome problems occur frequently, and there are some things that increase the risk of their happening. It is still not known why they happen. Down syndrome is a good example.

All cases of Down syndrome are caused by the presence of an extra chromosome 21. Ten percent of these are translocations (see discussion in Chapter 6). Ninety percent are new changes, unique to the affected child, that are caused by *nondisjunction*. This term is most easily understood by breaking it down: "junction" is a joining together, so "disjunction" is a taking apart. Normally, when the gametes are made, the pairs of chromosomes are split apart—the pairs are disjoined. This is the way it is supposed to happen. Eggs and sperm have half the normal number of chromosomes so that when fertilization happens, the zygote has the correct number again.

Nondisjunction is the lack of disjunction—it is the failure of the chromosomes in a pair to go their separate ways. As a result, an egg or sperm ends up with two copies of chromosome 21 instead of just one. When fertilization happens, the zygote then has three total copies of chromosome 21, which causes Down syndrome (Figure 7.1).

It is possible for nondisjunction to happen again in another pregnancy, but the risk is low. After it happens once, the chance of it happening

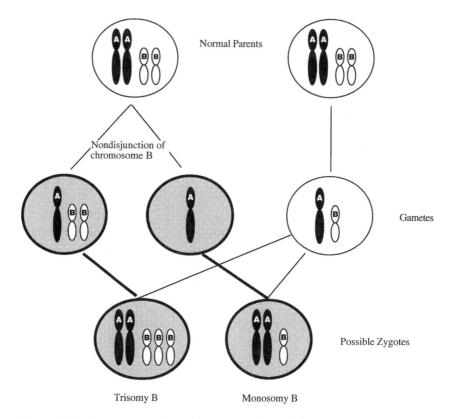

Normal Parents

Nondisjunction of chromosome B

Gametes

Possible Zygotes

Trisomy B   Monosomy B

Figure 7.1 Chromosomal nondisjunction. A and B are any two chromosomes. To simplify the figure, only these two chromosomes are shown. The other chromosomes should be considered normal. The abnormal gametes and zygotes are indicated by heavy lines and gray background. Both parents are normal. In meiosis—the process that makes an egg or sperm—the chromosome B pair fails to separate. As a result, two kinds of gametes are made. One has an extra B; the other is missing a B altogether. When the gametes fuse at conception, there are two possible outcomes: (1) Trisomy B—three copies of B. If this B is chromosome 21, this is Down syndrome. (2) Monosomy B—one copy of B. If this B is an X chromosome, this is Turner syndrome.

again is 1 in 100. This is the same as the risk to a woman at age thirty-five. You have probably heard that as women age their risk of having a child with a chromosome problem increases. This is called the "maternal age effect," and it relates to nondisjunction: as women get older, their risk of nondisjunction goes up. Thus, the risk for many chromosome problems (not just Down syndrome) increases as women age.

Nondisjunction can happen with any chromosome. It can cause there to be one too many or one too few chromosomes. People are most familiar with the nondisjunction problems of trisomy 13, trisomy 18, and trisomy 21. These are not the most common problems, they are just the most common that are seen in babies. These are the nondisjunction problems that are "mild" enough sometimes to allow a fetus to survive to birth. Most of the time, an abnormal chromosome number—including trisomies 13, 18, and 21—causes a miscarriage. Trisomy 13 and trisomy 18 are considered lethal conditions because most affected babies die before one year of age.

NEW MUTATION IN SEX-LINKED DISEASE

Sex-linked diseases are those that have their genes on the X or Y chromosome. They are discussed in greater detail in Chapter 13. In the past decade or so, our knowledge about these diseases has increased and the way we define them is somewhat in flux. It used to be that conditions were clearly "sex-linked recessive" or "sex-linked dominant." A recessive disease on the X chromosome would show up in males—who would not have a normal X to compensate—but not in females. It is recognized more and more now that "carrier" women—those who have one normal X and one X with a mutation—can have features of the condition. Sometimes the carrier women can be severely affected. So, the recessiveness of sex-linked disease is rather wishy-washy.

Statistically speaking, new sex-linked diseases usually happen because of new mutations. They do not tend to run in families undiscovered for generations. One-third of the time, the mutation happens in the egg that becomes an affected boy. Two-thirds of the time, the mutation happens in the sperm that becomes a carrier girl. The carrier probably will not be diagnosed but is at high risk of having an affected child (50% of sons or 25% of children overall). This one-third/two-thirds split is based on Haldane's method and is somewhat hypothetical. It works for some diseases (Duchenne muscular dystrophy) and not for others (hemophilia), but, while the ratios may be different, the idea is the same.[2]

When a boy is diagnosed with an X-linked condition, it may be appropriate to test the mother. It is good for her to know whether she is a carrier. It also may be important for her own health. Evaluation of the family pedigree may show other people—such as the mother's sisters—who are at risk to be carriers. Those people can be made aware of their risk and seek testing if they are interested.

The paternal age effect, mentioned above with dominant conditions, also increases the risk of mutations that can be passed by a daughter to a grandson (see Chapter 13, X-Linked Genes). Remember that men make two kinds of sperm—one with an X and one with a Y chromosome. The sperm of an older father can have new mutations on the X chromosome just as on any of the autosomes. Such a sperm would result in a carrier daughter and possibly affected grandsons.

MOTHER NATURE'S LEGACY

The most important thing to remember about new genetic disease in a family is that there is no "blame," no "responsibility." Changes in the genetic material happen all the time. Because of this we have good things, such as evolution and disease resistance. We also have bad things, such as birth defects and cancer. There is no way to predict a mutation or to prevent it. There is nothing that the pregnant woman or her mate does, or does not do, that causes a mutation to happen. Likewise, we have no control over what genes we pass on to our children.

There is quite a bit of lore, mythology, and superstition out there, but there is very little scientific evidence of anything. Some conclusions are easy: solar and lunar eclipses do not cause birth defects. Some conclusions are unavailable: there really is no evidence that illicit drug use causes defects, but it is not well studied.

8 Prenatal Testing

During pregnancy, a woman may undergo a variety of tests to monitor her health and that of the fetus. The most common fetal tests are the maternal serum biochemical screen and the ultrasound. Other tests may be done depending upon family history, maternal anxiety, and results of previous tests. Table 8.1 lists some common reasons that prenatal testing is recommended. This chapter will discuss the typical procedures and tests that can be done. For the sake of clarity, procedures are those actions taken to collect a sample—drawing blood, collecting amniotic fluid, and so on—and tests are the chemical or cellular analyses done on the sample. Table 8.2 is a brief list of the procedures, their risks, and the tests that can be performed on the sample.

Frequently, women will say that they do not want prenatal testing because they would not terminate a pregnancy. This assumes that the test result has some sort of decision-making power, which it does not. A test result is just a piece of information. It has no value and does not imply a particular action. The decision to test and the decision of what to do with the result are separate. If a test result is abnormal, there are many options. Yes, termination of pregnancy is one option. On the other hand, if the fetus is known to have a problem, special plans can be made for delivery at a hospital with the means to care for the baby. Choosing to avoid a test because a particular action is undesirable limits a woman's information about her pregnancy and her ability to care for herself, the fetus, and her family.

Table 8.1 Common Reasons for Prenatal Testing

General screening for the health and growth of the fetus
Monitor the fetus if the woman has a chronic or pregnancy-related health condition

Previous pregnancy with a birth defect or other problem
Family history of a birth defect or genetic disease
Parents are members of a high-risk ethnic group

Maternal age (risk of chromosome problems varies with maternal age)
Paternal age (risk of dominant genetic diseases varies with paternal age)
Maternal anxiety/parental wishes[a]

Use of artificial reproductive technologies

[a] The autonomy of the pregnant woman is always important but needs to be balanced with the risk of the procedure.

Table 8.2 Prenatal Procedures, Their Risks, and Tests That Can Be Done

Procedure	When it is done	What is tested	Benefits	Risks	Limits
Ultrasound	Anytime	Physical form of the fetus, growth	Not invasive.	Very low	Hard in obese women and when there is low amniotic fluid. May not see physically small things.
Maternal Serum Screening	15-20 weeks	Relative concentrations of chemicals in the mother's blood. Can suggest chromosome problem or breaks in the fetus' bodily integrity.	Minimally invasive to mom. Not invasive to fetus. Quick look for most common problems. Can suggest when more specific testing is needed.	Low[a]	Very indirect look at the fetus. Not a diagnostic test. Normal screening does not guarantee normal baby. Depends upon knowing the true gestational age.
Early Amniocentesis	12-14 weeks	Chromosomes, DNA, AFP	Nice compromise between CVS and routine amniocentesis.	Risk of spontaneous abortion ≤ 1%.[a]	Hard when there is low amniotic fluid.
Routine Amniocentesis	16-20 weeks or later	Chromosomes, DNA, AFP, fetal lung maturity	Technically easy, direct test of fetus.	Risk of spontaneous abortion ≤ 1%.[a]	Hard when there is low amniotic fluid.
Chorionic Villus Sampling (CVS)	10-13 weeks	Chromosomes, DNA	Done before pregnancy is socially noticeable.	Risk of spontaneous abortion ≤ 1%.[a] The placenta does not always have the same genetic make up as the fetus.	Does not test for breaks in bodily integrity (ex: spina bifida).
Percutaneous Umbilical Blood Sampling (PUBS)	18 weeks to delivery	Chromosomes, DNA, blood factors, anemia, infection	Can be used as treatment. Direct test of fetal blood.	Risk of spontaneous abortion 1-3%.[a]	Highest risk procedure. Hardest to do.

[a] Note: Risk of pain, bleeding, and infection are always present when a procedure involves a needle.

ULTRASOUND

Prenatal ultrasounds started in the 1960s and are now very common. In the developed world, almost every pregnant woman gets at least one ultrasound. These machines use high-frequency sound waves to take a picture or movie of the fetus. This is not an X ray—no radiation is used. Routine ultrasound is a noninvasive test—there are no needles. It is very low risk for both the pregnant woman and the fetus.

The "camera" part of an ultrasound machine is the transducer; this is a device about the size of a full tube of toothpaste or a telephone handset. It is placed against the abdomen. Sometimes it is necessary to put a transducer in the vagina, but this is not routine. The ultrasound works like sonar. It sends out sound waves and reads what bounces back. A computer turns the sound waves into a picture that is viewed on a television monitor. It looks like a grainy black-and-white movie. Liquid (such as amniotic fluid) absorbs sound waves and looks black on the machine's screen. More solid structures (such as bone) bounce back most of the sound waves, and these look white on the screen. Ultrasound works best when two structures of different solidity are next to each other.

There are two standard levels of ultrasound. A Level I or routine ultrasound is done to check for a heartbeat, monitor fetal growth and movement, and check the amount of amniotic fluid. A Level II or targeted or referral ultrasound is done if a problem is noted or suspected. The Level II is more detailed and/or concentrates on a particular structure or problem. There is also a fetal echocardiogram. This is a specialized ultrasound that looks at the fetal heart. This is done if a heart defect is suspected.

Ultrasound technology is really impressive today. A new type, the three-dimensional ultrasound, gives a result that can look like a regular photograph. Ultrasound does have its limits. It does not work as well when the mother is obese, when there is little amniotic fluid, or when there is more than one fetus. As with any test, the ultrasound only answers the question that is asked. For example, if the examination is of the fetal head and heart, the ultrasound will not necessarily see that there are missing fingers or toes. Also, ultrasound is not a good enough technology to see some types of birth defects, such as some heart defects, and it will never diagnose problems that are functional rather than structural: an ultrasound may find a structural problem of the brain, but it will not diagnose seizures.

MATERNAL SERUM SCREENING

Maternal serum screening, also called the "triple screen" (or "quad screen" if there are four things tested), is a very common prenatal test. The procedure is a simple collection of blood from the mother's arm vein. It is fast, moderately uncomfortable, and typically has no long-lasting side effects. There may be a number of different tests done on the blood sample to monitor the mother's health, such as a glucose level and check for anemia. The test done to look at the health of the fetus is the serum screen. It is also nicknamed the maternal serum alpha fetoprotein (MSAFP) test, although alpha fetoprotein is only one of the things measured. The most common compounds measured are alpha fetoprotein (AFP), estriol, human chorionic gonadotropin (Hcg), and inhibin. The concentrations of these compounds—both individually and relative to each other—can suggest a problem and indicate that more direct testing is needed.

Screening is a first look for something. It is not a final diagnostic test. It is intended to identify patients who need more evaluation. A Pap smear is a screening test, as is the blood pressure measurement taken during a routine doctor visit. If it is abnormal, you will be asked to return for more testing. Screening is never perfect. Some people at risk will be missed. Some healthy people will have an abnormal screening test. This is a consequence of the way screening tests are set up—it is not a failure of the test.

Alpha fetoprotein (AFP) is a protein made by the fetus. It is a small molecule that crosses the placental barrier. A measurable amount of it is normally found in the blood of a pregnant woman. Some problems in the fetus can cause a significant increase in the concentration of AFP in the mother's blood. Birth defects that disrupt the fetus's skin—such as spina bifida or abdominal wall defects—or the death of a fetus will result in high maternal serum AFP levels.

Estriol has been added to the maternal serum screening as a way to evaluate for trisomy 21 (Down syndrome). Human chorionic gonadotropin (hCG) is a hormone produced by the placenta and fetus. It is the compound measured in standard pregnancy tests. It has been noted that hCG is higher when the fetus has trisomy 21, so it is often part of serum screening.

An abnormal biochemical screen will prompt the obstetrician to recommend more direct testing of the fetus. Remember that the serum test is a screening test. Sometimes a screen will be abnormal when the fetus is actually fine. Sometimes a screen will be normal even though there is a problem with the fetus. Current maternal serum screening can detect

80–90% of cases with neural tube defects such as spina bifida and about 65% of trisomy 21 cases. Most women who have an abnormal serum screen go on to have normal ultrasound and/or amniocentesis.

AMNIOCENTESIS

Amniocentesis is most typically done around sixteen weeks gestation. There is an early version done between twelve and fourteen weeks in special circumstances. The early version has added risks. A long, thin needle is inserted through the mother's abdomen into the uterus. Ultrasound is used at the same time to help avoid poking the fetus with the needle. A tablespoon or two of fluid is removed and the needle is pulled out. The procedure itself takes one to two minutes.

Amniocentesis and the two tests described below, chorionic villus sampling and percutaneous umbilical blood sampling, are invasive tests that involve a needle. As such, they carry some risk to the woman and the fetus. Although these risks are low, it is important for a pregnant woman to be well informed about the procedures themselves. Table 8.3 lists some questions that might be asked by a woman of the obstetrician before consenting to the procedure.

Amniocentesis is the test with which most women are familiar. This procedure collects a sample of amniotic fluid—the liquid surrounding

Table 8.3   Questions to Ask Your Doctor Before the Procedure

How many of these procedures do you do in a week?
What is your complication rate?
What complications do you see in your patients?
What can I do to minimize my risk of complications?
What is this test likely to tell us?
When will test results be available?
How will you communicate test results to me?
How will the results of this test affect how you help take care of my pregnancy?
    If the result is normal
    If the result is abnormal
May I speak with another patient who has had the procedure?
May my husband/partner/support person be present?
How long does the procedure take?
What must I do to prepare for the procedure?
What must I watch for or do after the procedure?

the fetus. Amniotic fluid is, essentially, fetal urine. It contains fetal cells and biochemicals produced by the fetal kidneys, lungs, and other tissues. Various tests can be done on the amniotic fluid and the cells in it. This includes tests of chromosomes, DNA, the fetus's metabolism, and the same chemicals that can be tested in maternal serum.

Most frequently, amniocentesis is done to test the fetus's chromosomes. It should be remembered, however, that one is a procedure and the other is a test or analysis. Amniocentesis has a variety of uses. The amniocentesis procedure can also be done as a treatment—removing or adding to the amniotic fluid, for example. Later in gestation there are compounds in the amniotic fluid that indicate fetal lung maturity, so an amniocentesis may be done for this test.

CHORIONIC VILLUS SAMPLING

Chorionic villus sampling (CVS) is done between ten and thirteen weeks gestation. The instrument used is a long, flexible catheter. It is quite long but small in diameter, about 1.5 millimeters (1/16th inch). It is inserted into the uterus through the vagina (like a Pap smear procedure). The procedure can alternatively be performed through the mother's abdomen with a small needle. Guided with ultrasound, the catheter or needle is inserted into the placenta and a small amount of tissue is collected. The placenta does not have nerve endings, so the sampling itself is not painful; however, insertion of the instrument through the abdomen or vagina can be uncomfortable to painful. The procedure takes a few minutes.

CVS is a procedure done on the placenta. This is the earliest way to test a fetus after the pregnancy has started. It is most commonly done when the family history or the mother's personal history shows an abnormality or a risk of genetic disease. Women who get CVS are those with a significant risk of a problem and who want to know about it early in pregnancy. This way, if an abnormality is found, the pregnancy can be terminated before it is physically or socially obvious and while the termination is technically least risky.

CVS is most useful for examination of the fetus's chromosomes and DNA. For the most part, the placenta has the same chromosome makeup as the fetus (although this is not always true). It is a direct test and can be considered diagnostic of a problem if it is abnormal. It cannot test for spina bifida or for some other problems.

CVS carries a small risk of pain and infection, which is true whenever a catheter or needle is used in any procedure. There is also a risk of pregnancy loss. The miscarriage risk has been measured various ways, but generally it is about 1 chance in 100. This is roughly the same as the risk of amniocentesis. Obstetricians with more experience have lower complication rates: doctors who do more CVS procedures are generally better at it. When CVS has been suggested, there are some easy questions to ask. These questions are the same as those suggested for amniocentesis and are listed in Table 8.3.

CVS has been associated with limb abnormalities in the fetus—specifically missing fingers and toes. The earlier the CVS, the higher the risk. The highest risk was found with CVS done before 10 weeks gestation. After 10 weeks, the risk seems to be about 1 in 3,000, which is probably the natural risk for this birth defect. Limb defects are fairly common, and most of them happen in babies born to women who did not have a CVS procedure. Again, as technology and expertise advance, the risk will probably fall even further.

PERCUTANEOUS UMBILICAL BLOOD SAMPLING

Percutaneous umbilical blood sampling (PUBS) is a very invasive test that draws a sample of fetal blood from the umbilical cord. It is also called cordocentesis. It is performed after 18 weeks gestation but, as with amniocentesis, can be done earlier under high-risk circumstances. As with an amniocentesis, a needle is inserted through the pregnant woman's abdomen, into the uterus. Using ultrasound as a guide, the needle sticks the umbilical cord and draws blood out of the vein in the umbilical cord.

PUBS draws a blood sample. A frequent application is to measure fetal blood count looking for anemia. It is also possible to test for genetic diseases of the blood, such as hemophilia, and for some types of infections. PUBS is used therapeutically to give the fetus a blood transfusion if needed. A PUBS sample can be sent for a relatively rapid test of the chromosomes—faster than can be done on the cells collected by amniocentesis. This is valuable if a severe problem is suspected later in the second trimester and a woman wants the option of terminating an affected pregnancy before the legal time limit.

PUBS is slightly riskier than amniocentesis. The risk to the pregnancy is 1–3%, again with the most experienced persons having lower risks. It must also be remembered that PUBS is done only on the sickest or highest-risk fetuses: fetuses that are more likely to spontaneously abort whether the procedure is done or not.

PRENATAL TESTING IN CONTEXT

Pregnancy is not a disease, but it is a medical condition that should be monitored to maximize the health of both the mother and the fetus. There are two interesting social phenomena going on at the present time. On the one hand, some women are choosing not to have prenatal testing. They are of the mistaken belief that an abnormal test will require a particular action on their part. On the other hand, women are going to nonmedical ultrasound providers in shopping malls for a first "photo" of their child.

Perhaps it is the subjective difference between a test and a picture. Doing a test seems to imply that something bad will be found. Taking a picture is more a confirmation of normalcy. Testing is medical and harsh. Photographing is starting a scrapbook. By the second trimester, the majority of pregnancies will be normal and the babies born healthy. This is true regardless of whether one is getting a test or a picture.

9 What If a Test Is Positive?

Women and couples go into a pregnancy (planned or unplanned) generally assuming that everything will be fine. A good percentage of the time, they are right. If it never worked right, human beings would not have survived as a species. Unfortunately, things go wrong, too. As stated in the preceding chapter, some women assume that simply agreeing to prenatal testing obligates them to a particular action. It does not. This chapter discusses the major options available after a prenatal test is abnormal: (1) continuation of the pregnancy as planned and keeping the child; (2) termination of the pregnancy; and (3) continuation of the pregnancy and offering the infant for adoption.

It was mentioned in Chapter 1 that a geneticist will not tell someone whether or not to have a child. Likewise, a geneticist will be supportive of decisions a woman makes regarding her pregnancy. It is true, however, that experience is a good teacher. A geneticist has seen other families face the same decisions and has seen the outcomes of those decisions. There may be some assumptions made based on what other families have decided. These assumptions may or may not work for you. Please do not be offended. Remember that the doctor relies on you to share your thinking.

There are a few prenatally diagnosed conditions that can be treated during the pregnancy. These treatments are not cures—the baby will need further medication or surgery after birth. Some of these subsequent treatments are lifelong. Prenatal surgery for such birth defects as spina bifida, diaphragmatic hernia, and cleft lip receives a lot of press coverage, but it is still very experimental and very high risk. These will not be discussed further.

CONTINUATION AS PLANNED

After a prenatal test shows a problem, many women/couples choose to continue with parent and family plans that have already been made. However, maximizing the chances for successful pregnancy, delivery, and management of the baby may require some preparation. A fetus with a problem may require, for example, cesarean section delivery or surgery immediately after birth. Even when the long-term prognosis is good, it may depend upon what care the child gets in the first few hours or days of life.

A relatively common defect such as spina bifida is a good illustration. These children can do well but require attention starting before delivery. Spina bifida is relatively easy to diagnose during pregnancy by the maternal serum screen and/or ultrasound. Once diagnosed, plans are usually made for a cesarean section. This decreases trauma to the back and lets the doctor control delivery. Once born, the newborn is assessed for other problems and positioned to minimize trauma. If the spinal cord is open to the air, it can be covered and protected immediately. Neurosurgery is performed as soon as possible (usually in less than twenty-four hours) to close the opening, protect it from infection, and stop leakage of the cerebrospinal fluid.

If this child is diagnosed in utero, plans can be made to deliver the baby where all the above can be done easily. This is particularly important if the more appropriate hospital is in a distant city. Without prenatal diagnosis, valuable care and time are lost.

Sometimes a lethal condition is diagnosed during pregnancy. Anencephaly—failure of the skull and brain to form—or severe chromosome problems have a dismal prognosis. They are untreatable. In these instances, prenatal diagnosis can allow the parents to prepare for what little time they may have with the newborn. The labor and delivery ward, as well as the nursery, can be alerted not to be aggressive—no tubes or machines or needles. Thus, although the beginning of life and the end of life are close together, both passages may be taken with dignity and respect.

ELECTIVE ABORTION

In most of the Western world, women have the right to make autonomous decisions about their health care. These usually include decisions about continuing or terminating a pregnancy. As mentioned before, "abortion" is a general medical term that means the end of any pregnancy before 20 or 24 weeks gestation. This can be spontaneous (also called a miscarriage) or induced as a medical procedure. For clarity, this book uses "spontaneous abortion" to mean a miscarriage and "elective abortion" to mean the medical procedure.

Extensive legal, religious, and social debates surround the topic of elective abortion. These are beyond the scope of this book. The option of elective abortion is presented here because it is a legal and safe medical procedure that is sometimes an appropriate option. Whether it is the appropriate option for any reader is not the author's right to say.

Elective abortion is legal in all states of the United States until fetal viability. Laws vary from state to state, and the definition of viability varies as well. Medical viability means the ability of the fetus to survive separate from the mother. Science is pushing this point earlier and earlier, but an informally agreed age is 25 weeks gestation. (This itself is debatable, as 25 week fetuses are still very fragile and the vast majority of them either die or are disabled.) State legislatures take other things into account along with medicine when setting abortion law. So, by state laws, viability is most commonly defined as 20–24 weeks gestation.

In some states, minor women (up to age eighteen) may obtain an elective abortion only with the consent of a parent or the court. It is no longer required that married women have the written consent of their husbands. Laws concerning elective abortion are constantly changing — they will probably be different by the time this book is published. It is best to know the law as it applies to you.

There are a variety of procedures used to abort a pregnancy electively. There is one prescription medication, mifepristone (RU-486 or Mifeprex), which induces abortion. It is usually used in conjunction with other medications, such as methotrexate and misoprostol. It is widely used safely in Europe. It does have side effects of cramping, nausea, and vomiting. Use must be monitored by a health care professional. It can be used up to 9 weeks of gestation and is 95% effective. For those 5% of pregnancies not aborted by medication, surgical abortion is still an option. It should be recognized that methotrexate is a teratogen (see Chapter 4).

Use of the medication is low risk, low cost, and allows the woman to have more privacy and control. On the other hand, some women are not comfortable with the process of a medical elective abortion. In those situations, the medical option may not be useful.

There are different surgical procedures used for elective abortion.

Most involve inserting an instrument through the vagina into the uterus and removing the embryo/fetus and placenta. Different procedures are used depending upon the gestational age of the pregnancy. Some procedures that are safe for the pregnant woman in the early first trimester are less desirable in the later weeks. Since *Roe v. Wade* in 1973, elective abortions are performed by certified physicians in controlled, sterile, and safe conditions. Sedation and pain control is well used. Elective abortion procedures have a lower risk of complications for the pregnant woman than term labor and delivery.[1]

One method for elective abortion is induction of labor—exactly the same process used in normal term delivery. This is a longer procedure and usually involves admission to the hospital. In some situations, this may be the only option. When confronted with a fetal malformation or genetic disease, this method has one overwhelming advantage: it allows the geneticist or pathologist to examine the fetus directly. This is the single best way to determine what is wrong and estimate the chance of it happening again. This author has seen more than one family refuse an examination or autopsy and later come back with questions that cannot be answered because of that refusal.

ADOPTION

There is a third "pregnancy management" option that is not often mentioned: offering[2] a child for adoption. Unfortunately, this is often seen as a failing at something. Women are supposed to want the child they have carried in gestation. This is unfair to both the woman and the child. Sometimes the best thing is for someone else to be the parent. Adoption may be the appropriate option for a woman not comfortable with elective abortion or who does not have access to safe, legal, elective abortion facilities.

Certainly there are not always adoptive families available for severely disabled or malformed children. This is a larger societal problem that can be addressed elsewhere. Children with milder defects are more likely to find homes. Remember that a birth defect that may be overwhelming to one person can be a treatable inconvenience to another. There exists in the United States a network of families who will adopt a child with trisomy 21 (Down syndrome). After prenatal diagnosis of Down syndrome, contacting the local Down syndrome parent support group can get the ball rolling.

If a child with a birth defect or genetic condition is adopted out, it is important that the biological parents be told of any final diagnosis. Some conditions have a significant recurrence risk. The biological parents (and biological siblings) have the right to know their chance of having a similarly affected child in the next pregnancy. Likewise, the child and his or her adoptive family can benefit from knowing any genetic diagnoses that may arise in the biological family.

DECISIONS

When a fetus has a malformation or genetic disease, there are many things to think of and choices to make. The only wrong decision is the uninformed one. Each possible choice has medical, social, emotional, and financial consequences. It is imperative that decisions not be made rashly or for the wrong reasons.

PART III

Genetics in Infancy and Childhood

10 Abnormalities in the Fetus and Infant

Congenital anomalies are structural changes of the body that are present at birth. This is the fancy term for a birth defect. Depending on the anomaly, it may or may not actually be detectable during gestation or in the newborn period. This chapter will look at birth defects and genetic conditions that are likely to be diagnosed between conception and the first year of life. These anomalies fall into two general categories. The first are malformations: structural or anatomic problems. The second are dysfunctions: nonstructural or physiologic problems.

PROBLEMS OF STRUCTURE

These are the true "congenital anomalies." Three to five out of every one hundred newborns is born with some sort of anatomical difference. Some are of little consequence. Others are very serious. Antibiotics, vaccines, and general hygiene have controlled infections that once were the leading cause of illness and death. Children are safer now than they were before vaccinations, antibiotics, and flame-retardant clothing. As these other problems are controlled, genetics remains. Congenital anomalies and genetic disease are the most common cause of death to children younger than one year of age. Twenty-five percent (one out of every four) of admissions to pediatric hospitals is due to a genetic condition or congenital anomaly.

There are four types of congenital anomalies: malformations, dysplasias, deformations, and disruptions. The difference is the pathogenesis (how the problem develops). Malformations and dysplasias are caused by an intrinsically abnormal developmental process. *Malformations* are the commonly thought of birth defects. Organs or body parts are missing, in the wrong place, did not finish growing, or there are too many of something. (Sometimes the term "malformation" is used generically to mean any abnormality in the body. In this book it is used as specifically as possible.) *Dysplasias* are abnormal organizations of tissue in a single organ. The term "dysplasia" is a general medical term meaning "abnormal growth" and is also used to refer to cancers. A birth defect that is a dysplasia is not a cancer.

Deformations and disruptions happen when something external to the embryo or fetus impairs its growth and development. *Deformations* are abnormalities in the form or position of a body part because of mechanical forces. The head moulding that happens to all babies at birth is a deformation. Ears that are bent over or feet turned in because of constriction in the uterus are deformations. Most deformations correct on their own or with gentle manipulation of the involved body part. Some require more involved treatment. *Disruptions* are caused by a breakdown in normal development. These are usually more severe than deformations. Amniotic band sequence is a disruption. The amnion is the membrane sac holding the fetus and the amniotic fluid. Sometimes it can tear. There can be damage to the fetus from bits of amnion that wrap around hands, feet, or other body parts. Teratogens (see Chapter 5) cause disruptions because they are chemical agents or radiation that interfere with the growth of a normal fetus.

Some birth defects are diagnosed prenatally or right away after birth. They are obvious because they are easily visible or because they cause immediate problems. A cleft lip, missing leg, or defect in the spine can be diagnosed during pregnancy or in the delivery room. How quickly something is diagnosed does not always correspond with the seriousness. A cleft lip is evident immediately but is reparable with little or no long-term consequences. On the other hand, a blockage in the intestine may not be apparent for a few days but can be life threatening. Table 10.1 lists some structural birth defects and the various times of early life at which they are usually found. These are just a few examples, and the specific time of diagnosis varies from child to child.

It can be frightening and frustrating for a seemingly healthy baby suddenly to have life-threatening problems. Why didn't the doctor know before sending the newborn home in the first place? The answer is that there were no clues, nothing to suggest a problem. It is unrealistic (and logistically and financially impossible) to test every baby for every potential difficulty. Newborns have physical exams, weight checks, and

Table 10.1   Some Structural Birth Defects That Are Frequently Found at or Soon after Birth

Defect When Diagnosed[a]	Definition	Inheritance[b]	Treatment
Immediately			
Cleft Lip	Failed formation of the upper lip	Multifactorial	Surgery
Gastroschisis	Split in the abdominal wall, often with organs protruding	Multifactorial	Surgery
Limb Reduction	Missing all or part of a limb	Various	Prothesis, surgery, sometimes none needed.
Neural Tube Defect	Opening in the skull or spine, often with nervous tissue exposed	Multifactorial	Surgery. Will often also need treatment for hydrocephalus, club feet and incontinence.
Omphalocele	Large umbilical opening, often with organs protruding	Multifactorial	Surgery
Early			
Aortic Coarctation	Narrowing/stricture of the aorta	Multifactorial	Surgery
Choanal Atresia	Back of the nose is not open	Multifactorial	Surgery
Duodenal Atresia	Blockage of the small intestine	Multifactorial Common in Down syndrome	Surgery
Tetralogy of Fallot	Heart Defect Consisting of: pulmonic stenosis, thick right ventricle, ventricular septal defect, overriding aorta	Multifactorial Some with chromosome 22q11 deletion	Surgery. Often more than one surgery.
Late			
Horseshoe Kidney	Two kidneys joined together in the middle of the body	Multifactorial Common in Turner syndrome	Not correctable. Some patients may need surgery to adjust how the ureters leave the kidney.
Lobar Sequestration	Section of the lung that is not connected to the trachea	Multifactorial	Antibiotics for pneumonia. Surgery.
Poland Anomaly	Absence of pectoralis major muscle. Possible abnormalities of arm/hand	Multifactorial	Not correctable. Breast implant in females after puberty.
Tethered Spinal Cord	End of the spinal cord is anchored to the lower spine	Multifactorial	Surgery

[a] Immediate = easily diagnosed in the delivery room or nursery. Early = within the first week or two of life. Late = within the first year of life. Please note that these time scales are not absolutes.
[b] The most common inheritance pattern is listed.

blood tests. They are monitored for the most common and most dangerous things. Any peculiarity leads to more monitoring and testing. If there are no abnormalities in the common tests, and the baby does not have symptoms, no further evaluation is done. This is why a two-week checkup is so important. It is a chance for someone to double check that the newborn is adjusting well to the outside world.

Birth defects happen alone or in recognized combinations. When a baby has a single birth defect and no other problems, that defect is said to be an *isolated defect*. When there are combinations of birth defects, they are classified as syndromes, sequences, or associations. A *syndrome* is a collection of birth defects that are all caused by the same thing. For example, fetal alcohol syndrome includes a small head, poor growth, and distinct facial features. All of these things are caused by prenatal exposure to alcohol. Down syndrome is characterized by small ears, low muscle tone, short fingers and toes, a distinctive face, mental retardation, heart defects, and intestinal problems. All of these problems are caused by the presence of an extra chromosome 21, which is why this condition is also called trisomy 21.

A *sequence* is a series of birth defects that are causally related—one happens and it causes the next. A well-known sequence is Potter sequence. The primary problem is with the kidneys. They are malformed, function poorly, or are absent altogether. Because of this the fetus makes no urine. Amniotic fluid is mostly fetal urine, and if the fetus is not making any, there are secondary consequences. The fetus cannot move around as much, so the limbs become stiff. The face is compressed so that the baby looks like it is wearing a stocking over its head. Also, the lungs do not develop. "Breathing" amniotic fluid helps stimulate lung development. If there is no amniotic fluid, the lungs do not grow. When the baby is born, it usually dies soon because of the abnormal lungs. Potter is not a syndrome for two reasons. First, all of the defects do not have a common cause: they happen as a cascade. Second, there are many different reasons why the kidneys can be malformed or missing, so Potter is not a single entity. Some recognized sequences are as follows:

Potter: kidney dysplasia → decreased amniotic fluid → underdeveloped lungs, facial changes, stiff limbs

Pierre-Robin: small jaw → tongue is back and high → palate cannot close → cleft palate

Neural tube defect/spina bifida: neural tube closure fails → interrupted spinal cord → club feet, hydrocephalus

An *association* is a set of defects that is not a syndrome or a sequence but that happen together more than can be accounted for by chance alone. This is more of a statistical recognition that some combinations are more common than others. A common association is VATER (or VACTERL). The name is an acronym for the individual birth defects:

Vertebral anomalies
Anal atresia
Cardiac defects
Tracheo-
Esophageal fistula
Renal defects
Limb defects

Associations tend to be something of a wastebasket. It is best to make sure the defects are not due to a chromosome problem or other syndrome. For example, Holt-Oram syndrome has limb and heart defects but is caused by mutation in a single gene.

It is helpful to diagnose a syndrome, sequence, or association early. That way, tests can be done to find all the defects that might be present. Trisomy 21 is usually diagnosed right after birth. Children with trisomy 21 are at high risk for heart and intestinal problems. Doctors and nurses recognize the facial characteristics and other features of trisomy 21 and know to order other tests. These tests will be ordered even if the baby is not having any problems, just because it is known that the risk is high. There are other less common but equally recognizable syndromes that may be found in the nursery. Those syndromes that cause real problems in the newborn period will prompt monitoring and testing automatically. Serious structural birth defects may be found this way.

The genetic causes of structural birth defects vary. Isolated malformations are most commonly multifactorial, as was discussed in Chapter 3. Syndromes are caused by chromosome problems, and some are inherited in a dominant or recessive fashion. Malformations that occur in repeated patterns are more likely to be strictly genetic. Increasingly, the individual genes that cause structural birth defects are being found. At present, knowing the genes does not provide a treatment, but it can give good information about the chance of another child being affected with the same condition.

Some structural birth defects may not be found for months or years. Malformations of the breast or internal genitalia may not be found until puberty or until an infertility evaluation. Developmental delay and growth problems do not show up at all until some time has passed. Anomalies such as these are found because a problem arises or sometimes it is just coincidence. There are perfectly healthy people with an extra kidney or a small spinal abnormality. They do not even know they have these anomalies until, for example, they get a computed tomography (CT) scan after a car accident.

PROBLEMS OF FUNCTION

While still in the uterus, the fetus's metabolism is greatly supplemented by the mother. The mother's body supplies missing nutrients or eliminates built-up waste chemicals when the fetus's body cannot. This is over and above the normal support the mother's body provides. In some cases the mother's metabolism is making up for a significant deficit in the fetus.

Once the umbilical cord is cut, the baby's body must function on its own. Sometimes it does not. Human metabolism is a complex process with many steps that can malfunction. The basic idea of metabolic function and malfunction is demonstrated very simplistically in Figure 10.1. As with structural malformations, metabolic problems can show up at different times depending upon what is involved.

There is almost no metabolic problem that shows up in the delivery room. It takes at least a little time for the system to back up.[1] There are a handful of metabolic conditions that manifest fairly quickly—in one to three days after delivery. At about that time, an otherwise healthy newborn has what is euphemistically known as a "neonatal crash." They stop eating, become lethargic or irritable, and start to have heart and breathing problems. They get very sick very quickly. Analysis of the baby's blood will show a very high level of some chemical such as ammo-

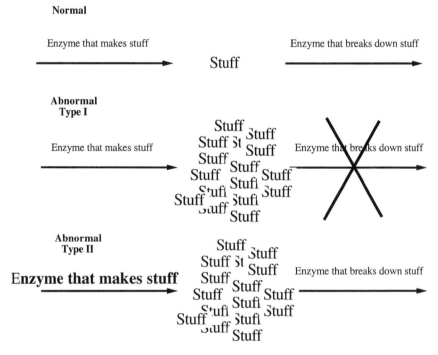

Figure 10.1 The basic problem of metabolic diseases. Normal metabolism consists of a series of chemical reactions that make and break down various materials in the cell. Abnormal metabolism consists, basically, of a block at one point, which causes material to build up behind it, or an excess of an enzyme, which creates more material than the cell can handle. In either case, the material accumulates inappropriately.

nia or lactic acid. These are normal by-products of metabolism that cannot be eliminated from the baby's abnormal body. Treatment starts to bring the levels back to normal while tests are run on the blood and urine. If a specific diagnosis can be made, treatment is then tailored appropriately. Unfortunately, there are still conditions for which no treatment is available. Fortunately, the most severe metabolic diseases are rare.

Some conditions are screened for by the state. This is the newborn screening or state screening or "PKU test." The goal of newborn screening is to identify disease so it can be treated before problems develop. All states screen for phenylketonuria (PKU). Otherwise, what is tested for varies from state to state. Diseases included in newborn screening include such things as galactosemia (problem metabolizing the sugar galactose), maple syrup urine disease (problem metabolizing certain amino acids), hemoglobin problems (such as sickle cell), and thyroid problems. Table 10.2 lists some conditions tested for by newborn screening, their frequency, the protein that is abnormal, and the symptoms.

The newborn screening diseases have the following things in common: (1) symptoms are delayed until after damage has already started; (2) they are relatively common in a large population; (3) there is a useful and fast test; and (4) there is a treatment that, if started early, can delay or eliminate the damage. Newborn screening is currently undergoing a revolution that will ultimately change the definition of it. At present, state testing is done because treatment is available. If current trends continue, testing will be done because easy and inexpensive testing is available.

There are some metabolic diseases that manifest early but that are not part of the newborn screening. They do not fit one of the above criteria: they are not common enough, there is not an easy test, or there is no useful treatment. Most often the early sign of a metabolic condition is developmental delay—failure of the child to sit, crawl, stand, or walk when expected. This can be tricky because there is a wide range of normal development. Sometimes the abnormality of body function shows up as something dramatic, such as seizures, failure to grow, prolonged jaundice, or chemical abnormalities in the blood. Since most of growth and development happens after the first year of life, this is discussed in more detail in the next chapter.

Other problems of function are not considered metabolic conditions (although, on a strict biochemical basis, they are) because they do not involve processing of nutrients or buildup of large compounds. Function can be lost because cells fail to form, die early, or cease to do what they

Table 10.2 Some Newborn Screening Diseases

Common Name	Abbreviation	Population Frequency	Abnormal protein[a]	Basic Problem
α_1-Antitrypsin Deficiency	AAT	1/8000	α_1-Antitrypsin (Also known as Protease Inhibitor 1)	Cells unable to repair damage. Liver problems, failure to grow. Later on can cause emphysema.
Biotinidase Deficiency	--	1/60,000	Biotinidase	Unable to make biotin, which is a cofactor for many proteins. Those proteins then cannot function. Developmental delay, hypotonia, seizures and acidosis.
Cystic Fibrosis	CF	1/2500	Cystic Fibrosis Transmembrane Regulator	Salts and water do not move as they should across membranes. Mucus is sticky. Harbors bacteria and impairs organ function.
Cystinuria	--	1/7000	Amino Acid Transporter 1 (has other names, too)	Kidney stones. Can lead to kidney failure.
Galactosemia	--	1/57,000	Galactose-1-phosphate	Unable to digest galactose (a part of lactose). Liver damage, neurologic problems, growth problems.
Hemoglobino-pathies (Sickle Cell, Thalassemia, etc)	Various: SS, SC, α-Thal, B-Thal	Varies	Hemoglobin	Abnormal structure of hemoglobin causes red cells to be fragile or oddly shaped. Anemia and tissue/organ damage.
Homocystinuria	--	1/200,00	Cystathione B-synthase	Homocystine accumulates. Neurologic damage.
Hypothyroidism	--	1/6000	N/A - Failure of the thyroid to develop	No thyroid function. Growth problems and mental retardation.
Maple Syrup Urine Disease	MSUD	1/200,00	α-ketoacyl-CoA decarboxylase	Unable to metabolize amnio acids leucine, isoleucine and valine. Growth and neurologic problems. Urine smells like burned sugar.
Phenylketonuria	PKU	1/12,000	Phenylalanine hydroxylase	Phenylalanine cannot be broken down. Growth and neurologic problems.

Note: Not all of these diseases are tested for in all states. Some states use the newer expanded screening outlined in the text.
[a] The protein listed is the most common defect for each disease. There are uncommon/rare forms of each disease caused by other protein malfunctions.

are supposed to do. Some metabolic conditions result from abnormalities of organelles—components of the cell. Abnormalities of mitochondria were mentioned in Chapter 6. These are metabolic conditions that result from impaired energy production in the cell.

EXPANDED NEWBORN SCREENING

Tandem mass spectrometry (MS/MS) is a relatively new technology used in the diagnosis of inborn errors of metabolism. Nationally, there is a movement toward using this technology for standard newborn screening. Some states are using this technology for all children, some are offering it to parents, and some are phasing it in. This trend is politically supported by the March of Dimes and various parent advocacy groups. Concerns have been raised by those who say that the technology does not have adequate specificity and sensitivity for large-scale population screening. It is one thing to test a specific patient but something completely different to test 1,000 babies a day. Individual physicians and websites offer MS/MS testing directly to parents. The cost for testing ranges but is generally between $35 and $50. Insurance coverage of this testing is variable.

One specific disease is driving the movement toward MS/MS screening: medium-chain acyl-coenzyme A dehydrogenase (MCAD) deficiency. This particular disease is important because it causes a type of sudden infant death syndrome (SIDS). Children with MCAD do not tolerate fasting, including short periods such as overnight. It is relatively easy to treat with frequent feedings and some diet supplementation. It is obvious that this particular disease has high priority for many people, particularly families who have already lost a child to the condition.

Conceptually, expanded newborn screening seems like a reasonable plan, but there are caveats. Parents and physicians requesting this expanded metabolic screen need to understand what it will and will not do. As with all other tests, there are benefits and disadvantages to this new process.

First of all, MS/MS will detect approximately thirty-five amino acid, organic acid, and fatty acid oxidation disorders. MS/MS is limited to a specific set of diseases. A normal MS/MS screen is not a guarantee of health because (1) as with any screening test, some children with a normal screening result will ultimately be found to have the condition, and (2) MS/MS can only evaluate those diseases testable by this method. It does not replace current screening methods for red blood cell problems (such as sickle cell anemia), hypothyroidism, biotinidase deficiency, adrenal hyperplasia (a hormone deficiency), or galactosemia.

Second, some conditions detected by MS/MS are treatable: PKU, MCAD deficiency, maple syrup urine disease, and citrullinemia among others. Unfortunately, MS/MS will also diagnose untreatable conditions such as nonketotic hyperglycinemia and propionic acidemia. These latter conditions lead to profound retardation and early mortality. Parents should be prepared for the possibility that MS/MS screening results will predict the early death of their child rather than provide them with a way to save its life.

Third, MS/MS diagnoses hereditary diseases. These diseases are inherited in an autosomal recessive fashion, and there will usually be no family history. A positive test means that both parents are carriers of the condition and that their other children are at risk for being carriers or being affected. When an MS/MS test is positive, genetic counseling is required and testing of other family members may be indicated. Parents must understand that testing their child may give them genetic information about themselves. (This is true for current newborn screening tests, too.)

Using MS/MS as a state screen raises quandaries among those who make public health decisions. One conflict is not new. Where is it best to spend limited dollars: extensive testing on all babies to diagnose perhaps a few more children a year, or making sure that all children receive immunizations? The machines themselves must be purchased and maintained. Increased numbers of abnormal screening tests will mean that more personnel are required to interpret and report the results. A larger system must be in place to contact and counsel parents and to retest the babies. This is not an impossible task, but it is a fiscal reality that must be faced.

The other difficulty is an ethical dilemma. The sensitivity of an MS/MS machine can be adjusted to report more or fewer results. This means that, while it is possible to diagnose something, a decision can been made by the state to do only tests 1 to 20 and not tests 21 to 35. Is it appropriate to knowingly restrict the amount of information that can be found? Does it make a difference if the tests not done are for untreatable conditions? Or the rarest conditions? What about having the machine do all the tests but only reporting the treatable conditions? These are not decisions that have been made by any state so far, but they are part of the discussion because a balance must be found between the ability to do the expanded newborn screening and the ability to support it with state dollars.

Physicians ordering the MS/MS screening should be prepared to discuss the limits of the technology, the possibility of diagnosing a lethal disorder, and the possibility of identifying nonpaternity or exposing parental health/genetic information. Parents need to understand what questions the screening will and will not answer and what will happen next if the screening comes back abnormal. Also, there needs to be a plan in place to refer families with positive screens to a geneticist for counseling and, as appropriate, treatment. More information about this technology and its use in newborn screening can be found in the following publications:

Tandem mass spectrometry for metabolic disease screening among new borns. MMWR. April 13, 2001;50(RR03):1–22 (Internet: http://www.cdc.gov/mmwr/preview/mmwrhtml/rr5003a1.htm)

Tandem mass spectrometry in newborn screening. ACMG/ASHG policy statement. Genetics in Medicine. July/August 2000;2(4):267–269 (Internet: http://www.acmg.net/resources/policies/pol-029.pdf)

ANATOMY AND PHYSIOLOGY

In problems of structure and function, the symptoms will depend upon the organ system involved. If the heart is structurally abnormal, or its metabolism is damaged, the result is heart failure. If the brain is malformed or the cells lose the ability to function, the result is developmental delay, mental retardation, or seizures.

At some point it can become difficult to separate disorders of structure from those of function. Obviously, if the heart has abnormal structure, it will not function correctly. The converse is also true. If the function of a cell or tissue is sufficiently impaired, it will start to change the organ's structure. Geneticists have historically divided the two types based on the idea that structural changes do not evolve over time while metabolic ones do. We recognize the superficiality of this division, especially in light of our growing genetic knowledge.

Structural birth defects can be inherited in any fashion: dominant, recessive, sex-linked, or multifactorial. The vast majority of genetic metabolic diseases are recessive. There is usually no family history except for, perhaps, an affected sibling. By definition, both parents are carriers of the condition, and the chance that they will have another child with the same thing is 25% or one chance in four. Mitochondrial conditions are inherited maternally. The risk of passing on a mitochondrial disease is statistically 50%, but in reality it is much more difficult to predict.

11 | Abnormalities in the Child

As children age, their chance of having a structural birth defect diminishes (but never disappears). Evaluation of a urinary tract infection at age six may show that there is only one kidney. Recurrent pneumonias to age ten may disclose that a part of the lung is not connected correctly. Sometimes the defect is the cause of the problem. Sometimes it is just a coincidence. Either way, structural malformations found at later ages are not immediately life threatening as they can be at birth. There may be the need for surgical correction or longer-term health consequences depending upon the organ involved.

In childhood, the problems that come to attention are those of growth and development. As in Chapter 10, these are essentially problems of structure and function. Growth is physical—gaining weight, height, and head size. Development is the learning of new things, adapting to the world. Abnormalities of growth and development can be caused by a variety of nongenetic things such as abuse, neglect, malnutrition, side effects of medication, and chronic illness. Discussion of these issues is beyond the scope of this book. This chapter will deal only with genetic causes of abnormal growth and development.

PROBLEMS OF GROWTH

One of my pediatrics professors had a saying: a child's most important job is to grow. When growth does not happen, something is not right. There are many genetic causes for failure to grow. They are broken down here into the two categories of failure to get larger (lack of height gain) and failure to thrive (lack of weight gain). There are also genetic syndromes of increased height or weight.

Short Stature

Some normal children are small because their normal parents are small. That is genetic, but it is not abnormal. Generalized failure to gain height is also called short stature. Pathologic (disease-related) short stature is a length or height less than 3% for age or a final adult height of less than 151 centimeters (59 inches) for females and less than 164 centimeters (64 inches) for males. There are dozens, perhaps hundreds, of conditions that cause short stature (Figure 11.1). There are also various ways to discuss these conditions—age of diagnosis, parts of the bone involved, inheritance pattern, and so on. The discussion here will be an overview only and will focus on the large divisions in type.

Short stature is divided generally into proportionate and disproportionate types. Persons with proportionate short stature have normal, if small, skeletal structure. Their arms, legs, trunk, and head are correctly sized relative to each other. Disproportionate short stature is caused by a skeletal problem either in the trunk or the limbs. All persons with significant short stature are correctly called dwarves whether they are proportionate or not. Another acceptable term is "little person." The term "midget" is considered inappropriate and offensive.

Proportionate dwarfism can be caused by a lack of growth hormone or its receptor. There are some genetic syndromes, such as 45,X (Turner syndrome), that have proportionate short stature as a primary feature. Prenatal exposure to alcohol and other teratogens also causes failure to grow. Proportionate dwarfism must be differentiated from true failure to thrive, which is discussed below.

Use of growth hormone to treat proportionately short children is controversial. When there is real growth hormone deficiency, giving it in shots does increase height significantly. In children with normal amounts of growth hormone, giving more increases growth velocity. It may increase final height by a few inches. This may be important if final natural height is disabling—too short to drive without assisting devices, for example. On the other hand, desiring to make a normal child a couple inches taller is really just cosmetic. It is quite a bit of money, time, and discomfort for a few inches. In patients with abnormal growth hormone receptors, giving growth hormone does effectively nothing. The body simply does not have the mechanism to recognize growth

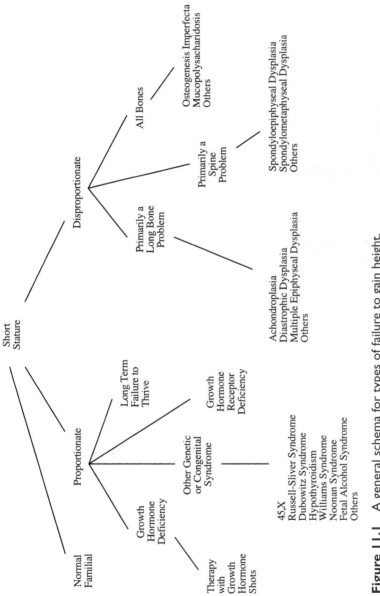

Figure 11.1 A general schema for types of failure to gain height.

hormone and has no way to use it. Growth hormone is not given to people whose bones are mature, because the only effects it has after maturity are disfiguring.

Disproportionate dwarfism happens in 1 in 4,000 to 5,000 live births and results from a primary bone problem—a skeletal dysplasia. There are many of these conditions. Achondroplasia is the most common type of skeletal dysplasia. Persons with achondroplasia have abnormal growth of their long bones—the arms and legs—with relatively normal growth of the skull and ribcage. Other skeletal dysplasias cause abnormalities of the spine while leaving the arms and legs more normal. There are also problems such as osteogenesis imperfecta ("brittle bone disease") that affect all the bones.

The quick way to categorize short stature is by comparing the upper and lower halves of the body. The center point is the pubic bone. The body's upper segment is from the top of the head to the pubic bone. The lower segment is from the pubic bone down. In children older than nine with normal height or proportionate short stature, these measures are roughly equal—the upper segment/lower segment ratio is one.[1] Ratios greater than one mean that the legs are short. Ratios less than one mean that the problem disproportionately affects the skull and spine.

X rays of the various bones always give helpful information. One common X ray test is a measurement of bone age. This is done by taking an X ray of the hand (in babies, it may be an X ray of the whole body). Bones are all present at birth, but some of them are still mostly cartilage, so they do not show up on X ray. As a person ages, the bones become denser. This change happens in a predictable pattern. By comparing a child's X ray against a normal standard, it is possible to determine how mature the bones are. Whether a bone age is advanced or delayed can be another clue to diagnosis.

Failure to Thrive

Failure to thrive starts out as simple failure to gain weight. In the longer term, failure to thrive may also mean failure to develop. Social deprivation and abuse can cause failure to thrive. Likewise, chronic illness such as HIV infection or cancer can prevent a child from growing and thriving. These causes are important but will not be discussed here.

Genetic failure to thrive can be divided into four categories: (1) structural problems that interfere with feeding; (2) functional problems that interfere with feeding; (3) inability to absorb calories and nutrients; and (4) increased calorie need. Table 11.1 lists some examples. It is

Table 11.1   Categories of Failure to Thrive—Genetic Diseases and Birth Defects

Structural problems interfering with feeding	Functional problems interfering with feeding	Inability to absorb or use calories	Increased calorie requirement
Short tongue	Brain malfunctions	Galactosemia	Cystic fibrosis
Cleft palate	Hypothyroidism	Adrenal insufficiency	Nephrotic syndrome
Nasal obstruction	Sucking/swallowing malfunction	Diabetes Mellitus	Congenital heart disease
Esophageal atresia	Ornithine Transcarbamylase Deficiency	Insulin receptor deficiency	Cancer
Pyloric stenosis	Congenital myotonic dystrophy	Mucopolysaccharidosis	Any disease that increases metabolism
Intestinal atresias	Prader-Willi Syndrome[a]	Biliary atresia	Epidermolysis Bullosa

Table modified from Kirkland RT. Failure to thrive. In: Oski FA, DeAngelis CD, Feigin RD, McMillan JA, Warshaw JB, eds. *Principles and Practice of Pediatrics*. Philadelphia: Lippincott; 1994:1050.

[a] Although Prader-Willi syndrome causes obesity in childhood, newborns and infants with it have severe hypotonia and feeding problems.

important to discover the underlying problem because treatments differ. If a child has a cleft palate, that structural problem makes it hard to suck on a bottle. Use of special nipples and repair of the cleft lead to normal feeding and good weight gain. This is very different from the child with cystic fibrosis who can eat, chew, and swallow easily but whose body cannot digest food well and who has an increased caloric need because of a stressed metabolism.

Tall Stature

Too much growth is also a problem. There are some conditions that lead to tall stature or obesity. Tall stature is length or height more than 98% for age and sex. In adult males, it is height over 192 centimeters (76 inches). In adult females, tall stature is height over 179 centimeters (69 inches).

Marfan syndrome is one condition with which people are familiar. President Abraham Lincoln is thought by some to have had Marfan syndrome (this is not proven). People with Marfan syndrome have tall stature and are loose jointed. They also can have problems with their heart and large blood vessels. Marfan syndrome is a problem with the protein fibrillin, which is found in the connective tissue—the stuff between the cells. There are other genetic conditions that cause abnormally tall stature.

People with these conditions are said to have "marfanoid" features because Marfan syndrome is the paradigm for these conditions.

Some tall stature diseases also have mental retardation or metabolic problems. Fragile X syndrome is the most common heritable cause of mental retardation. One of the features of this condition is a large habitus—not just height but also bulk. Homocystinuria is a metabolic disease. Some states test for homocystinuria in their newborn screening programs (see Chapter 10). It looks just like Marfan syndrome, but there is mental retardation and a vitamin or diet treatment.

There is a set of conditions called overgrowth syndromes. These are typically genetic diseases that cause large body size in infants and children. Adult size often is not remarkable. Childhood motor development can be delayed because the muscles are doing more work to move the larger body. The long-term prognosis depends on the condition. Infants of diabetic mothers are usually large because the amount of sugar in the mother's blood stream causes excess growth of the baby. These babies start to "even out" once their own metabolism takes over.

Isolated overgrowth of a limb or organ is called hemihypertrophy or hemihyperplasia ("half overgrowth"). This can be part of a genetic syndrome or can be a single problem. Hemihyperplasia can be difficult to manage because surgical reduction does not always work. There is an association between hemihyperplasia and some types of cancer, so it is important for children with this condition to be monitored. There are two things to keep in mind. First, everyone is a little asymmetric. Small differences in size from one side to the other are expected. Second, when there is significant asymmetry, both sides should be evaluated because it is not necessarily the large side that is the abnormal one.

Obesity is mentioned here as a growth problem although it is, theoretically, controllable. Some genetic syndromes often have obesity as a component. The most well known of these is Prader-Willi syndrome. In this condition eating is a compulsion and there is never a sense of satiety. Affected persons suffer from severe weight problems and associated health issues.

PROBLEMS OF DEVELOPMENT

There are two ways to think about problems of development—delay in achieving milestones, and loss of milestones already achieved. A developmental milestone is what it sounds like: learning to do something that is a basic function of living. Smiling back, reaching for objects, sitting, standing, walking, climbing stairs, being toilet trained, and so on, are developmental milestones. Milestones normally happen in a predictable sequence that coincides with nervous system maturation.

Development is typically measured in four areas: gross motor (sitting, walking, running, riding a bicycle), fine motor (manipulating toys, feeding oneself, drawing), language (understanding and expressing words), and social adaptation (play, sharing, cooperating, taking turns). Minor variations among children are expected. Girls tend to progress faster in language and social areas. Boys master the gross motor milestones a bit earlier. Some children skip steps—such as going from sitting to walking without ever crawling. It is all fine as long as development progresses at a reasonable pace and there is no persistent weakness in a particular area.

Delayed development is the lack of progression—not learning milestones in the first place, or learning them much later than expected. The child who is exclusively right-handed to the point of never using the left side at all has a specific type of gross and fine motor delay. A child who walks and runs but cannot follow simple commands by two years of age has a language delay. As precise as these descriptions are, they do not by themselves indicate a specific diagnosis. Children with any sort of delay will need a thorough evaluation.

For example, a child who is not using one arm may have a simple, common, acute condition like a dislocated elbow (nursemaid's elbow). That child may have a more serious problem with the brain or nervous system, with the musculature in or the circulation to that arm. The abnormality may just involve the arm, or it may be part of a larger syndrome. The child may have had a stroke due to a genetic disease that causes abnormal blood clotting. In such a case, the primary problem is actually a blood disease, even though what the parents notice is absence of use of an arm. Figuring out the diagnosis even of a relatively simple problem can become complex fairly quickly.

Language is an interesting situation because there are many nuances. A child can be delayed in language simply by growing up in a bilingual household. This is an observed phenomenon. Presumably, learning two words and sets of syntax for everything delays initial language comprehension, although it is beneficial in the long run. Otherwise, the most common reason that children do not develop language is that they cannot hear. The first evaluation done on any child with a language delay is often a hearing test. However, there are many reasons for deafness. Some are genetic and some are not. Determining the reason for hearing loss is important because treatments differ.

Some states have started neonatal hearing screening. This is like the newborn metabolic screening discussed in Chapter 10. Babies get a quick, painless hearing test in the hospital. If it is abnormal, they are sent for a more thorough test. If that is abnormal, they can be referred for treatment right away. If hearing aids or surgery are appropriate, this can be done early—before language development. Sign language can be started early as needed. Either way, identifying a hearing problem as young as possible increases the child's chances of learning language in a developmentally appropriate fashion.

Children with birth defects may have developmental delay even though they are mentally normal. For instance, a child born with only one hand will have to learn to compensate, and some fine motor skills will be late or missing. Spina bifida causes incontinence, so toilet training will be a problem. Allowances are made for these obstacles.

Loss of milestones is a separate developmental problem. In this situation, a child who had previously mastered something loses the ability to do it. For example, an eighteen-month-old becomes unable to walk. As with delayed development, this may indicate a reparable physical problem. However, "loss of milestones" as a diagnosis is first associated with a specific set of metabolic genetic diseases. These are called storage diseases because they result from accumulation of material in the cell.

Storage diseases are classified by what is stored or by which part of the cell is involved. Glycogen storage diseases are, logically enough, those conditions in which the molecule glycogen accumulates in the cell. Glycogen is a component of fats and fat-like compounds. In lysosomal storage diseases, any of a number of products can build up, but the problem starts in the lysosome. The lysosome is one of the organelles. It is a bag of enzymes that function in very acidic (low pH) conditions. Its primary function is to rid the cell of bacteria and harmful compounds.

Different storage diseases affect different parts of the body. Some only affect muscle, others affect nerves. Some include changes in the eye, such as cataracts. In others, a substance may collect in all the cells of the body. Those that cause loss of developmental milestones most often have some material that builds up in the cells of the central nervous system. The material stored is a normal by-product of metabolism that the body is unable to break down. The product itself may be toxic or, more often, the accumulation becomes so great that the cell ceases to function.

Individual storage diseases are uncommon to rare, but there are a number of them. Altogether, they occur once in every 1,000 to 5,000 live births. The vast majority, like all metabolic diseases, are autosomal recessive. Some are X-linked. Treatments are starting to be available for some of the lysosomal storage diseases, such as Gaucher, Fabry, and

Hurler (mucopolysaccharidosis I) disease. Using an intravenous infusion, patients are given the enzyme that their bodies lack. Conceptually it is like giving insulin to a diabetic. Over time, the stored material breaks down and the symptoms improve. Treatment is lifelong.

FIRST SIGNS OF A PROBLEM

Abnormalities in growth and development are common in children. There are many underlying causes, and correct diagnosis is important. Dividing these problems into distinct categories is somewhat artificial. Both the symptoms and their causes overlap. By itself, growth failure is not a diagnosis: it is a symptom or a sign. Failure to grow in weight or length may be the first clue to an underlying problem. A child who does not gain weight may be normally small, may have a growth hormone problem, or may be affected by a metabolic disease.

There is normal variation in how children grow and learn new tasks. Parents of twins see this most distinctly. No two youngsters are exactly alike in their development. The difficulty comes in determining whether a particular deviation is really a problem or just "little Suzie's way of doing things." It can be useful to know the average age by which a child should have learned a task. It is better to know how late is too late. If there are serious questions, testing can be done by the pediatrician or a developmental specialist.

12 When the Problem Cannot Be Fixed

When a pregnancy is diagnosed, there is expectation for the future and it is generally positive. Future parents understandably expect the stereotype: a normal pregnancy and delivery followed by all the joys and frustrations of having a new baby. There is also, consciously or unconsciously, an imagined future of first steps, first words, going off to school, graduations, weddings, and grandchildren. And honest folk admit to the occasional negatives, such as the first fender bender, broken hearts, a failed class, college hangovers, and lost jobs.

Unfortunately, some families have to deal with hospitalizations, medical technology, multiple doctors, and the early death of a child. This chapter will consider some of the decisions such families may have to face. Chapter 9 was about managing pregnancy after an abnormal test. This is the next step. What issues must be considered after a child is diagnosed with a chronic or even a fatal condition?

GIVING AND GETTING BAD NEWS

There is simply no universal gentle way to give or get bad news. Even when there is suspicion of a problem, having the doctor confirm it can be devastating. Likewise, health care providers cannot always predict how a family will react to the information. Those who give bad news a lot are probably better at it than those who do not, but no one is perfect. Unfortunately, some care decisions must be made right away. A family that has just heard something they did not expect may be asked immediately what they want done. Ideally, there is time. Frequently, there is not.

When training medical students and residents to give bad news, I tell them to pick three pieces of information about the child. These three things are what the parents need to hear the most strongly. They may be bad or good, immediate or future. The discussion is not limited to these three things, but they are what matters most. For example, telling a family that their new baby has trisomy 21 may include these three things: the diagnosis, the immediate health of the child, and the need (or lack of need) for surgery. A condition that is less well known may require more directed information: the diagnosis, the major complication of this diagnosis (mental retardation, short stature, and so on), and the predicted longevity. Each situation is very much unique.

Depending upon the family's state of mind, the discussion may end with these three things. It may be followed by some standard genetic information or with an extended period of answering family questions. Whatever the first talk involves, it should always be followed up soon by other sessions. Not only do future sessions reiterate and remind, they also allow for new information depending upon the baby's status and a chance to answer more questions. When a baby is sick and diagnostic tests are continuing, the picture can change quickly. New information can seem to contradict what was known the day before.

Doctors do not always know what a family needs, so there is an extended network of nurses, counselors, clergy, social workers, and others who may be involved. Even with all these people available, the family still needs to communicate its needs. It is OK to ask the same questions again. It is OK to ask for help. It is OK not to put on a brave face.

TALKING TO THE CHILD

Very young children who are mentally normal may not understand the seriousness of their illness, but they may know that something is wrong. Certainly they are experiencing the pain of needles, restrictions on their behavior, and the emotions of their parents. Babies and toddlers mostly need reassurance that they are loved and that they are not alone. Older children may have questions about sickness and death.

It is wrong to assume that a child is ignorant of what is happening. Keeping an illness, or the seriousness of an illness, from a child is impossible. They know that their friends do not have to go to the hospital, or have surgeries, or eat a special diet. They may overhear conversations. They can learn to read signs on clinic doors. They may even be told things by well-meaning adults who have no idea about the child's level of understanding. Both healthy and sick children interact with many people every day. Not everyone can be in on the secret.

The best way to control how your child learns something is to tell it yourself. It does not have to be a science lecture. It does not even need to happen all at once. It does, however, have to be honest, factual, and age-appropriate. Children have questions that can be very simple or amazingly profound. If there is no answer to a question, then "I do not know" becomes the answer.

On the other hand, imagination can be worse than reality. Your child may believe that he or she is going to die when all that may happen is a broken bone. A child may believe that something he or she did caused the illness or that it is a punishment. Our culture is full of unfortunate phrases such as "only the good die young" and "it's the will of God." Talking to your child not only lets him or her know what you are thinking, it also lets you know what your child is thinking.

TALKING TO SIBLINGS

When children learn that their brother or sister has a problem, they have many questions. Some of these questions may be the same that the parents have: How and why did this happen? Is it going to get better? Other questions are unique to a child's point of view. The answers to these questions do not need to be complex, and, as with the sick child, they do need to be age-appropriate.

Babies born with visible birth defects may look like they have been violently injured somehow. It is important to explain that the cleft lip, or missing hand, or spina bifida does not hurt. It is not an injury, it is just the way the new baby was put together. Along the same lines, the sibling may wonder whether the same thing will happen to them. Younger children are not thinking about reproduction—their chance of having an affected child. They are thinking about the chance that they are going to wake up some morning and have the same thing that the newborn does. The answer to this question is easy but needs to be said specifically: no, you will not look like this someday.

Young children also believe in magical thinking. If a child does not want a younger sibling, and then the newborn is sick or dies, the child may think that his or her wishes are responsible for the parents' sadness. Again, it is important to state the obvious: nothing you did or thought caused this to happen.

When one child is diagnosed with something genetic and heritable, it may be necessary to test siblings for the same thing. The need for a blood test can be handled with the same explanation useful for vaccinations: this will hurt for a minute, but the goal is for you to be healthy. The advent of topical anesthetic cream has improved this experience for both children and adults. When the test comes back, normal or abnormal, share the results with the child. A normal test can be greeted with "Hey! We proved you're healthy." An abnormal test will need some explanation, such as "We need to give you the same help we're giving your sister." More specific answers to the child's questions may need the help of your pediatrician or other medical specialist.

As siblings get older, they will ask questions requiring advanced answers. Since more and more genetics is being covered in school, they may be exposed to a family condition through a textbook. They will want to know at an adult level how their own health or that of their future children may be affected. There is no specific age at which these questions need to be addressed. In general, they need to be answered as they are asked. The more sophisticated questions may need the help of a pediatrician or geneticist. It is completely reasonable to make an appointment just to answer a young person's questions.

SHORT-TERM VERSUS LONG-TERM CONSEQUENCES

All medical decisions have a short-term consequence and a long-term one. Each decision is part of a larger string (or flood, or avalanche) of treatment options. It can be very difficult to grasp where a particular decision falls. Some choices are fairly easy and obvious. A child born with an isolated cleft lip or an extra finger will need to be seen by a surgeon very soon. The decision is whether or not to have surgery to repair the cleft or take off the finger. The immediate consequence is that the baby will have surgery, with its known risks. The long-term consequence is that the baby will grow and develop and be unaffected as an adult.

Other decisions are harder. A severely affected infant will die soon without some procedure—surgery or mechanical ventilation or an experimental drug. If the procedure is done, the infant may die anyway. If the infant survives, he or she will be severely impaired and will never be mentally or physically normal. The decision is whether or not to do the procedure. The short-term consequence is that the procedure has a chance of prolonging the infant's life. The long-term consequence is that doing the procedure will not correct the underlying cause of the problem and it may prolong suffering.

One thing that must be remembered is that some severely affected infants do not die right away. Parents can be caught believing that a child will die soon after birth only to find themselves with a severely affected family member for months or years. A woman may have decided not to terminate a pregnancy with the mistaken understanding that the baby would miscarry or be stillborn. The anecdotes one most often hears are of families who feel "blessed" to have had their special child. There are also families who feel burdened, even betrayed by that child.

Health care providers see some things families often miss. The long-term consequences of having a child with special needs are not only medical: they are also social, financial, and emotional. This is true even when money is not an issue and there is a strong support network of friends and relatives. Early short-term decisions will affect longer-term choices, such as keeping or changing jobs, sending other children to public or private school, and where to live. Many families juggle this rather well. Others struggle all the time. Most are probably somewhere in between.

On the other hand, health care providers also have a better feel for good outcomes. Some conditions that are shocking at birth are actually rather straightforward to manage. Even though it may mean surgery, a lifelong drug, or a hearing aid, the child ultimately does very well. Parents can be overwhelmed by the amount of things they are told they have to do: medicines, doctor visits, special diets, splints, and so on. In these instances, it may be important for the family to hear that by the time the child is sixteen the biggest worry will be whether he or she really can be trusted with car keys.

MEDICAL FUTILITY

At the beginning of the twentieth century, doctors could do relatively little. Their role was more as comforter. Wars, epidemics, and increasing technology changed medicine in the following hundred years. By the last quarter of the century, the comfort level with technology became so high that both patients and doctors used it routinely. The use of machines was no longer an enhancement: it was an expectation. This is the "technological imperative" of medicine—because we have a machine, we must use a machine. Believing in technology so much has led to the idea that not using a device must mean neglecting the patient.

The technological imperative is not true. Machines are tools to be used only when they are medically appropriate. Definitions of medical appropriateness vary, but doctors, other health care workers, and families are beginning to understand that technology is not a miracle. In the 1990s, medical ethicists—professionals who wrestle with the dilemmas of medicine—began to advocate the medical futility movement. Essentially, this is the opposite of the technological imperative. More realistically, it is a moving back to the idea that caring for someone humanely does not always mean using technology. This dilemma reflects on the previous section about short-term and long-term consequences.

We now have common machines that can keep lungs breathing and hearts beating and can substitute for kidneys. In this way, a person's body can be kept going for some period of time. But if there is no likelihood of cure or improvement, use of the technology is futile. Sometimes the most humane thing is to withhold or withdraw the technology and let the patient die. Doctors are often accused of wanting to play god. But technology has become the new God in medicine.

Another myth is that machines can never be turned off—once a device is used, its use must be continued. Withdrawing a machine such as a ventilator or dialysis can be a very difficult decision. Ethically and legally, however, withdrawing and withholding in the first place are the same thing. It is the same as stopping a medicine that is not working or has bad side effects.

HOSPICE

The modern hospice program began in England in the 1960s under the direction of Dr. Cicely Saunders. The goal was and is compassionate care for the dying with adequate use of pain medications and other comfort measures. Put another way, hospice advances the sanctity of life by nurturing its quality rather than its quantity. The best outcome may be thought of as a chance to die comfortably in one's sleep, preferably at home.

Hospice is viewed by some as a last resort, or a giving up. It is not. Hospice is an active program of care and treatment. It just does not buy into the technological imperative—it does not invoke that God. Interestingly enough, patients in hospice may actually survive a bit longer than if they stayed in an aggressive medical program because their pain and stress are better addressed. Table 12.1 lists some of the myths and facts about hospice.

According to the Hospice Foundation of America (http: // www. hospicefoundation.org), 80% of hospice can be done at home. Hospice facilities are available, and programs vary from city to city. It is team-oriented and deals with all aspects of disease, death, and dying—the

Table 12.1   Myths and Facts about Hospice

Myth: Hospice is where you go when there is "nothing else to be done."

Reality: Hospice is the "something more" that can be done for the patient and the family when the illness cannot be cured. It is a concept based on comfort-oriented care. Referral into hospice is a movement into another mode of therapy, which may be more appropriate for terminal care.

Myth: Families should be isolated from a dying patient.

Reality: Hospice staff believe that when family members (including children) experience the dying process in a caring environment, it helps counteract the fear of their own mortality and the mortality of their loved one.

Myth: Hospice care is more expensive.

Reality: Studies have shown hospice care to be no more costly. Frequently it is less expensive than conventional care during the last six months of life. Less high-cost technology is used, and family, friends, and volunteers provide 90% of the day-to-day patient care at home.

Myth: You cannot keep you own doctor if you enter hospice.

Reality: Hospice physicians work closely with your doctor of choice to determine a plan of care.

From the Hospice Foundation of America: http://www.hospicefoundation.org/what_is/myths.htm

emotional, social, and spiritual as well as the medical. Patients enter hospice when they are diagnosed with a terminal illness and the decision is made to change care plans. The entire family and network of care-givers are supported by hospice.

Some local programs have limited space, so they take on new patients based on prognosis, such as having six or fewer months to live. Patients in such programs are not let go if they have not died in six months. Some children taken on as babies may still be in a hospice program as teenagers. This is further indication that hospice is not a place or a treatment regimen but a concept of care.

THINGS TO THINK ABOUT

Doctors and nurses, social workers, and clergy tend to be caught in dilemmas. They do not want the family to despair, but they also want to be honest. They want to give a patient every reasonable chance, but they do not want to be inhumane. They want to respect the family's autonomy, but they recognize that some things just cannot be done.

The families have burdens also. Parents need to communicate with each other and agree on courses of action. They should understand as much as possible and ask questions when there are unknowns. Probably the hardest thing is that parents and families need to try and see the consequences— both immediate and long term—of their various decisions.

The families that seem to be the most comfortable in this uncomfortable situation are those that can separate their emotional turmoil from the business of medical decision making. In such families that I have encountered, the baby was diagnosed early with a terminal condition. The parents were not shy about showing their grief or asking for help, but when it came to making hard decisions they were led by their heads rather than their hearts. They gathered the information they needed, learned the benefits and risks around each decision, and understood the difference between the situation right now and the potential situation in the future.

PART IV

Genetics in Puberty and Adolescence

13 When Things Go Right

We all change as we grow and age. Childhood and puberty are times of rapid change. Genetic problems can affect pubertal development. Some of these problems will be discussed in the following chapters. In this chapter will be a brief overview of normal male and female puberty. The discussion begins with a description of *sex-linked* inheritance. Although many of these genes play no direct part in sexual maturation, sex-linked diseases manifest differently between the sexes.

SEX-LINKED INHERITANCE

Sex-linked genes are those found on the X and Y chromosomes. They are thus "linked" to a sex chromosome. Sex-linked diseases often affect males and females differently. This is because females have two X chromosomes and males have an X and a Y. Sex-linked diseases are to be differentiated from sex-limited diseases. *Sex-limited* conditions affect only one sex because of the anatomy or physiology unique to that sex. For example, only men get prostate cancer and only women can have uterine fibroids.

X-Linked Genes

The trick to understanding X-linked genes is to remember that how a disease manifests depends upon the number of X chromosomes present. Most X-linked diseases are recessive: the presence of a normal gene decreases or prevents disease symptoms. Males have only one X, so they can inherit an abnormal gene without any normal counterpart. For this reason, X-linked diseases are more common in males. Figure 13.1 shows a typical X-linked pedigree. The pedigree clue that it is not an autosomal dominant condition with incomplete penetrance is that there is no male-to-male transmission—the abnormality never passes directly from father to son. This is a soft indication, but it can be a good place to start. Women who have to be harboring the mutation but who do not show symptoms are obligate carriers. Once a mutation is found in a female, or she manifests the phenotype, she is a confirmed carrier.

Use of the term "carrier" here is difficult. It is easy when a woman has a mutation but no symptoms. When a woman has a mutation and symptoms, she is called a "manifesting carrier." This is terminology used almost exclusively for X-linked diseases. When disease shows up in someone who has one normal and one mutated gene on any other chromosome, the disease is called dominant instead of recessive. The way we think about X-linked diseases is starting to change, but the old terminology is still in use.

Figures 13.2 and 13.3 show the typical inheritance patterns for an

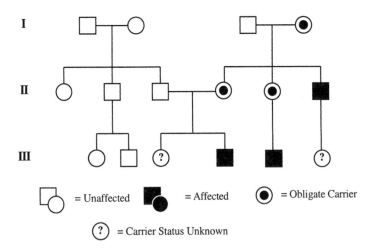

Figure 13.1 Typical pedigree of X-linked inheritance. Affected persons are all blood-related. Note that the disease appears in more than one generation and only in males. There is no transmission from father to son (which is impossible in X-linked conditions). See Figures 6.1 and 6.7 for comparison. Spouses were not all drawn in the interest of space. Please refer to Figure 2.2 for an explanation of the symbols. An obligate carrier is a woman who, because of her position in the pedigree, must have the mutation.

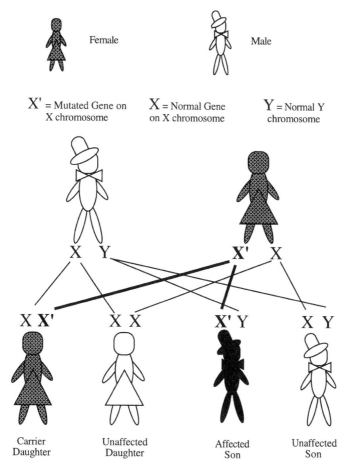

Figure 13.2 X-linked inheritance, mother a carrier.

X-linked condition. Note that the risk of passing a condition on depends upon the sex of the affected parent. If a woman carries an X-linked condition, one of her X chromosomes is normal and the other has a mutation. If she passes the normal X, the child, boy or girl, is normal. If she passes the mutated X, a boy will be affected and daughters will be carriers. For any pregnancy, the chances of any outcome are as follows: affected son, 25% (1 in 4); carrier daughter, 25% (1 in 4); unaffected son, 25% (1 in 4); noncarrier, unaffected daughter, 25% (1 in 4).

The affected sons are *hemizygous* for a mutation. This term is specific for X-linked genes. It means that, in an otherwise normal state, there is only one allele of a gene present. The term hemizygous works in males

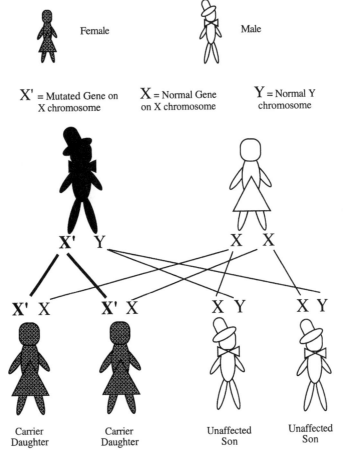

Figure 13.3   X-linked inheritance, father affected.

for most genes on the X and the Y: they are hemizygous for normal genes or mutated genes on the X. In the clinical setting, hemizygosity only matters when there is a mutation. There are some genes on the tip ends of X and Y that are on both chromosomes—these genes have two alleles in both males and females.

When a father is affected by an X-linked disease (is hemizygous), he can pass the mutation only to his daughters. His sons get the father's Y chromosomes. That's why they are boys. The sons get a normal X from their mother, so they do not have the condition that affects the father. All of the daughters will be carriers. They can only get the father's mutated X. They also get one of the mother's normal X chromosomes.

Now comes the difficult part(!). Sometimes women can have symptoms of the disease. Rarely, a woman has both alleles mutated. She is therefore homozygous for the mutation and manifests the condition. That is straightforward recessive inheritance (see Chapters 6 and 7). There are also two special circumstances under which a woman can show an X-linked recessive disease: Turner syndrome and unfortunate Lyonization.

Chromosome disorders were covered in Chapters 6 and 7. Turner syndrome is the condition in which a person has only one sex chromosome, an X chromosome. Women with Turner syndrome can manifest an X-linked disorder for the same reason that males do: they are hemizygous for the mutation. Although they are female, they only have one X. If that X chromosome has a mutation, there is no normal allele to take up the slack and they have the disease.

In women with the normal complement of two X chromosomes, there is a process called Lyonization: in every cell of the body, one of the X chromosomes is inactive. On the inactive X, a large percentage of the genes are chemically altered so that they are not transcribed. This process is called Lyonization after Dr. Mary Lyon, who first described it in 1961. Inactivation is controlled by a gene called XIST (pronounced "exist") that is close to the centromere on Xq. When the XIST is active, that chromosome is turned off. From cell to cell, the inactivation is random. This is a normal process.

Sometimes the random inactivation turns off a normal gene in a tissue affected by the abnormal gene. Remember, if the abnormal gene causes a skin problem but it is only active in the liver, it does not matter. If, however, it is active in the skin, the disease manifests. This is unfortunate Lyonization. When it happens, the recessive X-linked condition shows up. The woman with the one mutated X is then a manifesting carrier. It is impossible to predict whether this will happen. When it does happen, it is very difficult to know how severe the disease will be.

There are a few X-linked diseases that are considered dominant. They are usually also lethal in males. In women who have one normal X and one mutated X, the disease manifests completely (has full penetrance). Specific symptoms may differ among patients (variable expressivity) (see Appendix B). Some of the variable expressivity is due to Lyonization. Males who inherit the mutated X have no counterbalancing normal allele and typically do not survive to birth. The males most often spontaneously abort. When a male survives, it may be because that male has two X chromosomes in addition to the Y. This is designated 47,XXY and is a condition called Klinefelter syndrome. Sometimes somatic mutation can cause an X-linked lethal disease in a surviving male.

X-linked inheritance can be confusing because there are so many exceptions. Attention must be paid to the sex of both the parent and the child. X-linked diseases are always more severe in males and in females with Turner syndrome. Female carriers can manifest the condition.

Y-Linked Genes

There are few genes on the Y chromosome. The most important is the Testis-Determining Factor (TDF), which drives male development. Without this gene, the embryo develops as a female. The gene is found close to the upper end of the Y chromosome (distal Yp). Sometimes, recombination between the X and Y chromosomes can move this gene to the X. TDF is a single gene. It is like all other genes in that it can have mutations or be missing. These situations will be discussed in Chapter 15.

Y-linked inheritance is much more straightforward than X-linked inheritance. A man passes his Y chromosome to all his sons and never to his daughters. So, a man affected with a Y-linked condition will have no affected daughters and 100% affected sons (Figure 13.4). Although not a disease, the easy example is "maleness." A man passes this condition to all his sons but to none of his daughters.

NORMAL SEXUAL DEVELOPMENT

Genetic sex is set at conception. The human embryo gets either an X or a Y in the sperm. From conception to 11 weeks after, the sexes are physically indistinguishable. At 11 weeks, if TDF is present, testes form and cause the fetus to develop as a male. In the absence of TDF, the fetus develops as a female. Once the anatomy is in place, it is static through birth until puberty. These are the primary sexual characteristics—the presence of female or male genitalia.

Pubertal development is a very complex process. Those readers interested in the biochemical, hormonal, or psychosocial aspects should refer to other sources. The remainder of this chapter is devoted to the structural changes that take place during puberty in females and males. This is also called the development of secondary sexual characteristics. These changes are classified into stages first described by Dr. J. M. Tanner in 1976. We refer to sexual development in puberty as Tanner stages or sexual maturity ratings. They range from Tanner 1 (prepubertal) to Tanner 5 (fully mature). Stages are specified for body parts: pubic hair, breast, and genital. Table 13.1 lists the stages for each. Generally, the stages occur in a predictable pattern; however, some variation is fine. Pubertal

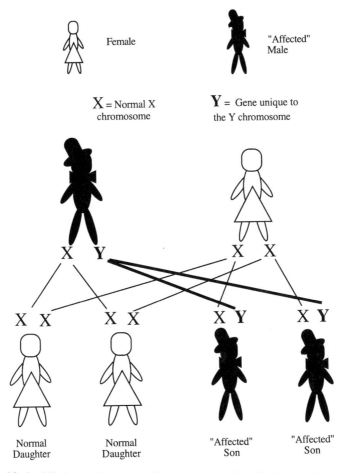

Figure 13.4 Y-linked inheritance. The sons are called "affected" (in quotation marks) because many of the genes on the Y are unique to that chromosome. Thus, some normal things are Y-linked.

development and growth are adversely affected by malnutrition. Some medications, particularly male and female hormones, can affect puberty.

In girls, the first sign of puberty is breast enlargement. This happens on average at 10 years of age but can be as early as 8 or as late as 13 and still be normal. Growth of pubic hair can start at the same time. The peak growth spurt occurs about a year after the beginning of puberty. Growth is mostly complete by the time menstruation begins. Fat deposition increases and lean muscle mass decreases. Internally, the uterus and ovaries increase in size five to seven times.

Table 13.1   Tanner Stages or Sexual Maturity Ratings

Stage	Female		Male	
	Breast	**Pubic Hair**	**Genitals**	**Pubic Hair**
1	Prepubertal	None	Prepubertal Testes <2cm length	None
2	Areola widens and darkens. Breast bud underneath	Sparse, long, slightly pigmented hair on labia or pubic area	Testes >2 cm, <3.2 cm. Scrotum enlarges and darkens	Sparse, long, slightly pigmented hair at base of penis or scrotum
3	Breast enlargement	Increased quantity, curliness, coarseness and pigmentation of hair	Testes >3.3 cm, <4.0 cm. More enlargement and thinning of scrotum. Linear growth of penis	Increased quantity, curliness, coarseness and pigmentation of hair
4	Further breast enlargement with mounding of areola above breast	Curled, coarse hair covering anterior pubic area	Testes >4.1 cm, <4.9 cm. Scrotum changes continue. Penis increases in all dimensions.	Curled, coarse hair covering anterior pubic area
5	Adult	Adult covering anterior pubic area and inner thighs	Adult. Testes >5 cm. Scrotum dark and thick. Penis adult size and configuration.	Adult covering anterior pubic area and inner thighs
6				Extension of hair growth up line to umbilicus

In boys, puberty starts with testicular enlargement and, on average, starts a year later than in girls. The average age for boys is 11 years, with a normal range of age from 9 to 14. During puberty males have a greater growth velocity than females—they grow taller, faster. The male growth spurt happens about 2 years after the beginning of genital enlargement. Males have increased lean muscle mass as an effect of testosterone. The penis roughly doubles in size.

Some normal features of puberty can be distressing, such as gynecomastia (breast enlargement) in males and increased facial and body hair in females. In extreme cases, evaluation for underlying medical conditions may be indicated. Treatment can be undertaken if the problem is severe or distressing enough.

SUMMARY

There are genes on the X and Y chromosomes. All of these genes, by definition, are sex-linked even though they may have nothing to do with sexual development or function. Unlike autosomal genes, the risk of passing on or inheriting a sex-linked disease depends upon the sex of both the parent and the child. Sexual development is very complex. It can be monitored in part by following the sex-specific Tanner stages that describe pubertal development.

14 When Things Go Wrong—Female

Abnormalities of female sexual development can happen prenatally or at puberty. Abnormal prenatal development results in birth defects— structural problems of primary sexual characteristics. Even if primary structures are normal, aberration in secondary sexual characteristics may become apparent at puberty. Sometimes external structures are normal and mature normally but internal genitalia are abnormal. Technically, these are birth defects even if they are not found until later in life.

BIRTH

External Genitalia

At birth a baby girl's genitalia can look unusually large and dark. This can be a normal reaction to maternal hormones. If so, the changes will resolve as the baby's body gets rid of the hormones.

When the genitalia are truly abnormal, they are called ambiguous: it is not possible to tell just by looking whether a baby is female or male. When the baby is genetically female, it means that the genitalia are masculinized—made to look more male. Masculinization happens because the female fetus is exposed to abnormally high levels of male hormones. These hormones can come to the fetus through the mother's body or they may be produced by the fetus itself.

All women have some androgens ("male" hormones) in their systems. If the mother has a medical condition in which her body produces abnormally high levels of androgens, this can affect the fetus. Some women take medications that contain androgens or that act like them. These can adversely affect development of female genitalia in the fetus.

Occasionally the fetus itself has a genetic or metabolic problem that causes high androgen levels. The most common of these is a type of congenital adrenal hyperplasia (CAH) caused by deficiency of the enzyme 21-hydroxylase. This condition is included in the newborn screening of some states. In addition to the masculinization of female genitalia, CAH also causes salt and sugar imbalances in the body. It can be life threatening, but it is treatable. There are other, rarer, causes of female ambiguous genitalia. Some are hormone problems. Others are genetic problems of primary organ development.

The genital abnormalities can be corrected surgically in most cases. The ability of a surgeon to bring the genitalia all the way to normal female depends upon the degree of malformation. Correction of external genitalia may or may not coincide with some correction of internal genitalia. Also, correction of external genitalia alone will not correct infertility. There are some malformations of the genitalia that can be fixed and that do not affect fertility. This question is best discussed for each affected child individually.

When there are external abnormalities for any reason, two questions must be answered. First, what is the genetic sex of the baby? This will be answered with a chromosome test. Chromosomes are discussed in Chapter 5. Chromosome problems are reviewed in Chapters 6 and 7.

The second question is about the internal genitalia structure. Is it present or absent? If present, it is normal or abnormal? The most common test done to answer this question is an ultrasound. More detailed testing may be done with an MRI. Occasionally a surgeon will perform an exam under anesthesia—a direct look at the structures using fiber optics or other technology inserted into the urethra or vagina. It is done under anesthesia because it is uncomfortable, but it is not surgery. It is, essentially, a detailed pelvic exam.

At the end of a medical evaluation, the following things should be known: the genetic sex of the baby, external and internal genitalia structure, presence or absence of gonads, and any associated medical problems. Diagnosis of the underlying problems, treatment decisions, and prognosis can then be decided.

Breast

As with the external genitalia, infant breasts can respond to mother's hormones. This can cause mild enlargement of breast buds under the nipple. These usually regress within six months. There can also be a colostrum-like discharge from the nipples that occurs in the first week of life. Supernumerary (extra) nipples are very common—up to 5% of the population—and are found in both males and females. Full extra breasts are less common but do happen. There are various genetic conditions that cause underdevelopment or complete absence of breast and nipples.

One common malformation affecting the breast is called Poland anomaly. The usual finding is absence of the pectoralis major muscle on one side of the chest. This is the muscle that can be felt on the front of the chest right at the armpit. (Hold the fold of skin in front of the armpit between your finger and thumb. The muscle you feel is the pectoralis major.) In addition to the absent muscle, there can be abnormalities of the breast, arm, and hand on that side. The breast and nipple can be small or completely absent. It should be remembered that normal women have asymmetric breasts. The breast on the side of the dominant hand is usually slightly smaller. This is normal asymmetry and is not Poland anomaly.

PUBERTY

As already mentioned, pubertal development is complex. It would be impossible to cover every potential abnormality. Here we will discuss two specific problems—Turner syndrome and androgen insensitivity syndrome (AIS). For the sake of example, the classic, textbook presentations of these diseases are used. For both conditions there is a range of features. In Turner syndrome (45,X) the primary sexual characteristics are normal but maturity is impaired. In AIS the primary structures, particularly the internal ones, are abnormal but puberty progresses as expected.

Turner Syndrome—45,X

Turner syndrome is the clinical entity that happens when one of the sex chromosomes is missing. Usually the sperm that contributes to the embryo is missing either the X or the Y. The chance of having a baby with Turner syndrome does not change with the mother's age; however, Turner syndrome is very common at conception and is a frequent cause of spontaneous abortions.

At birth there may be physical features suggesting this diagnosis. The genitalia are normal female, but there are other findings, such as a wide neck and swollen hands and feet. Coarctation of the aorta—a narrowing of the large blood vessel coming out of the heart—is associated with Turner syndrome and may be discovered soon after birth. On the other hand, Turner syndrome is increasingly diagnosed in mildly affected females when there are problems with puberty or infertility. These are people who, as babies, appeared normal. There is nothing in their health history to suggest the diagnosis until they fail to have periods or have difficulty conceiving a pregnancy.

Women with Turner syndrome have a uterus, although it may be small. Their ovaries are present but are very abnormal. They are often referred to as streak ovaries because they are a smudge of tissue instead of a fully formed, round compact organ. (Normal ovaries are about the size and shape of an almond still in the shell.) Because the ovaries are dysfunctional, the normal hormone surges at puberty cannot happen. Secondary sexual characteristics do not develop as expected. Delay in puberty or late/absent onset of menstruation may be what prompts the genetic evaluation.

Hormone therapy can help move a patient through puberty. Growth hormone has been approved for the treatment of short stature in Turner syndrome. Severe underdevelopment of breasts can be treated surgically with implants. There are even cases of artificially conceived and assisted pregnancies in women with Turner syndrome.

Females with Turner syndrome can be mentally retarded, but many are intellectually fine. There can be some learning disabilities. Turner syndrome women seem to have specific problems with visual-spatial tasks. Otherwise, I am aware of women with Turner syndrome who are doctors, nurses, and other professionals.

Androgen Insensitivity Syndrome—AIS

This condition used to be called testicular feminization. Now that the specific biochemical problem is known, the name has changed. Androgen insensitivity syndrome is caused by a mutation in the androgen receptor gene, which is on the X chromosome. It is inherited in an X-linked recessive fashion (see Chapter 13). This means that female persons with two X chromosomes do not show features, but males, who are hemizygous, are affected. It may help to refer back to Figures 13.1 and 13.2.

When discussing this particular condition, it is easy to become confused. In affected persons the genetic sex (genotype 46,XY) does not match the phenotypic sex (they are female). For simplicity, genetic sex will be referred to as XX or XY and phenotypic sex as male or female.

Figure 14.1 shows how this condition is inherited and how it manifests. Compare with Figure 13.2. The difference is in the phenotypic sex of the offspring. XX people are unaffected and female. XY people are unaffected and male. X′X people are unaffected carriers and are female. X′Y people are affected and are **female**. Their chromosomes and their features are different from each other.

It is important to remember that all the other genes are working. This includes the Testis-Determining Factor (TDF) gene on the Y chromosome. Women affected with AIS have TDF. Therefore, they have testes. The testes function normally in producing testosterone and other

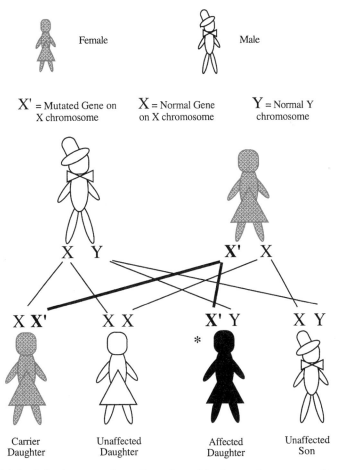

Figure 14.1   Inheritance and manifestation of Androgen Insensitivity Syndrome. Note that the affected daughter (marked with an asterisk) has an XY genetic sex even though she is female.

hormones. The problem is that some of these androgens have no way to influence the way parts of the body grow. The cell protein that normally responds to these hormones is not functional. To use an old analogy, the body is making plenty of functional keys (hormone) but the locks (receptors) are all broken.

The testes make a variety of hormones that do a variety of things. Except for testosterone and its action in cells with the androgen receptor, the hormones work as expected. Müllerian-inhibiting factor (MIF) is another hormone made by the testes. It works just fine and its receptors are functional. The consequence of MIF function is that embryonic development of the uterus, upper vagina, and fallopian tubes is suppressed. This is a normal function of this normal hormone. People with AIS, therefore, do not have these organs. Testosterone also influences such things as muscle mass and metabolism. Since different receptors are involved, these processes go forward with "male" programming. In spite of this, the outward appearance of persons with full AIS is that of a typical female.

So, in AIS the internal organs and metabolism are abnormal, but at puberty there is normal female maturation—except that menstruation never starts. The breasts enlarge, pubic hair grows, height increases, body proportions—narrow waist, wide hips—are female. Unless an earlier abdominal exam shows the presence of testes or the absence of a uterus, these women are not diagnosed until there are questions about fertility.

The only medical problem faced by women with AIS is that the testes have to be removed. There is a risk of cancer. Normal testes are outside the body, where it is cooler. In women with AIS the testes are in the abdomen, where it is warm. They do not produce sperm because of this environment, and there is a chance that they will grow abnormally and become malignant. Once they are removed, the risk is eliminated.

GIRLS INTERRUPTED

There are two stages of sexual development. Primary development is the formation of the genitalia. This happens in the embryo during the first trimester. Secondary development is what happens at puberty. The primary anatomy is acted on by hormones. The body changes and grows in a relatively predictable pattern.

Abnormalities in female sexual development can involve the internal genitalia, external genitalia, or both. There can be primary malformation of the genitalia or breast. There can be failure of the secondary sexual characteristics to mature at puberty. The specific conditions discussed here—congenital adrenal hyperplasia, Turner syndrome, and androgen insensitivity syndrome—are the most common examples. There are, however, quite a few genetic, metabolic, and hormonal diseases that interfere with normal primary and secondary female development.

15 When Things Go Wrong — Male

As with females, male sexual development can have primary malformations or secondary problems with maturation or both. Unlike females, males do not normally have internal genitalia. All male genitalia are visible outside the body. This makes problems more obvious, and so they are usually diagnosed earlier than puberty. Also unlike females, the male urinary system and genital system do not fully separate during development. A single abnormality thus can affect two different organ systems in the male.

BIRTH

Penis

There are two problems of the penis that can be seen at birth: micropenis and hypospadias. Micropenis is a small penis. Hypospadias is a penis in which the urethral opening is underneath rather than on the end. Hypospadias is fairly common as birth defects go and is thought to be increasing in frequency.

A normal penis in a term male is 3.5 centimeters long (1 3/8 inches). There is a range of normal. A baby is said to have a micropenis if it is less than 2.5 centimeters (1 inch) at birth. Sometimes the penis is surrounded by fat on the pubic area, which can make it look short, but that is not a micropenis. That is a buried or hidden penis. This may require surgical correction, but the penis is otherwise normal. Micropenis is caused by abnormally low levels of androgens or an insensitivity to androgen (see Chapter 14 for a discussion of androgen insensitivity syndrome). It is also found in some specific genetic conditions, such as Prader-Willi syndrome and trisomy 21.

Hypospadias occurs in about 3 out of every 1,000 males born. The urethra—the tube through which urine and semen exit the body—is displaced from the end. Specifically, it is found on the undersurface of the penis somewhere. This may be as far forward as the glans or as far back as behind the scrotum. If the urethra is only displaced a small amount, hypospadias may not be diagnosed until circumcision. (An opening on the top of the penis is epispadias—a different and much more rare condition.)

There is some suggestion that the incidence of hypospadias is increasing, possibly due to an increase in hormone-like substances in food and water. Hypospadias is also increased in males conceived using a technology called intracytoplasmic sperm injection to treat the infertility of their fathers. The incidence of hypospadias varies with ethnic group, being significantly lower in Hispanics.

Mild hypospadias, called distal or first-degree hypospadias, may be a cosmetic problem only. Correction is surgical and can usually be accomplished in a single procedure. Correction can be done whether or not the baby has been circumcised. Previously, males found to have hypospadias were not circumcised because it provided tissue for surgery. Newer techniques have made this less important. If there are any questions, though, it is easiest to put off the circumcision until the hypospadias correction surgery.

More severe hypospadias is often associated with other problems, particularly urinary tract malformations and ambiguous genitalia. When the urethral opening is on the shaft of the penis, that is second-degree hypospadias. In third-degree hypospadias, the opening is on the scrotum or behind the scrotum. These forms are harder to correct, especially if there are other malformations in the area. Also, the more severe the hypospadias, the more likely there is to be an underlying syndrome causing it. If this is the case, then there will be other medical issues that must be addressed.

Fortunately, correction of hypospadias is not an urgent procedure. Babies who are not yet toilet trained can be allowed to grow for a while. This makes the surgery both safer for the child and technically easier for the surgeon. There are debates about when such surgery is best done. Current standard practice has the aim of completing genital surgery before sexual awareness in the child—before the child starts to understand that he or she is a boy or a girl. Children with severe hypospadias used to be raised as girls, even if they were genetic males. This is much less common now. It is more typical to reconstruct abnormal genitalia based upon the genetic sex of the child.

Testicles

The testicles start out in the abdomen and then descend into the scrotum with later embryonic and fetal development. Both testicles normally descend into the scrotum between 35 and 40 weeks gestation. Since testicles retract up against the body when it is cold, baby boys are best examined when they are warm and relaxed.

Two or three out of every one hundred baby boys (2–3%) have at least one undescended testicle. This percentage rises with prematurity. Seventy-five percent of the time, the testicle will descend on its own by three months of age. Sometimes human chorionic gonadotrophin (hCG) or testosterone injections are given, and these help stimulate the testicle to move. Occasionally surgery is necessary to complete the descent. It is important to bring the testicle out of the abdomen because there is an increased risk of cancer if it is left there. Mammalian testes function normally when they are slightly cooler than core body temperature.

If it is a simple, unilateral undescended testicle, then the prognosis is excellent both for health and fertility. If both testicles are undescended in a term baby, that is more complex and suggests that there may be an underlying problem. Sometimes there are related malformations, such as a hernia or a testicle that is small and underdeveloped. Rarely, the testicle is completely absent. Because the urinary system is connected, there are kidney problems in some males with undescended testicles, usually when both testicles are involved.

PUBERTY

Male puberty, on average, starts a year later than in females. It is as complex as in females and equally fraught with emotional and psychosocial concerns. One normal variation that can be distressing is gynecomastia (breast development) in males. This happens between Tanner stages 2 and 3 of sexual maturity and can last for two years. Often it regresses by itself, but it can be treated with medication or surgery when it is significant. Some medications and drugs of abuse (including alcohol) can cause gynecomastia. There are genetic and hormonal problems that can also be involved. Any suggestion that breast enlargement in a male is not "just a normal part of puberty" should be evaluated.

Boys with external genital malformations are identified before puberty. There are no "hidden" genitalia, as there can be with girls, so it is less likely that a boy will proceed through puberty before a problem is discovered. There are cases of early puberty in boys, which are largely caused by hormone-producing tumors. There are some rare single-gene problems that may affect puberty in otherwise normal males. A common genetic cause of delayed puberty in males is Klinefelter syndrome.

Klinefelter Syndrome—47,XXY

Klinefelter syndrome results from having an imbalance of sex chromosomes when there is at least one Y present. Usually this is one Y and two X chromosomes, but there can be more of each. The *aneuploidy*— abnormal chromosome number—results from nondisjunction, the failure of chromosomes to separate when egg or sperm are made. About half the time the problem is in the making of the egg. The other half of the time it is the sperm that is abnormal. There is an increased risk of having a male with Klinefelter syndrome as mothers get older, but not as much as with Down syndrome (trisomy 21).

At birth, males with an extra X chromosome appear normal. Their primary sexual characteristics are present and unambiguously male. Occasionally, 47,XXY will be discovered before birth because of an amniocentesis. The pregnancy may have been tested because of a problem or simply because of maternal age and routine screening abnormalities.

Most males with 47,XXY have normal intelligence, but many have minor learning disabilities or delays in development. It is common for Klinefelter syndrome to be discovered only because of abnormal puberty or adult infertility. The testicles are small and do not enlarge as expected. They also do not function normally. Klinefelter syndrome is essentially a problem of testicular failure. The other secondary sexual characteristics, such as body hair, penile growth, and voice changes, are decreased because the testicles are not making normal amounts of hormones. Most men with Klinefelter syndrome are also infertile because the testicles make little or no sperm.

Just as women have some androgens, men have some estrogens— female hormones. In Klinefelter syndrome the level of estrogen is high relative to that of androgen. The result is that some "female" characteristics develop. Specifically, about half of Klinefelter males at puberty may develop breasts, they have more body fat (less lean body mass), and can have a more female body shape. Affected males tend to be taller than the average for their families.

Testosterone injections are used to assist puberty. The hormones promote virilization (male appearance), which can promote a more positive self-image. Regular treatment can also increase the libido; however, the infertility is not corrected by androgen injections. Breast enlargement can be treated surgically.

As with Turner syndrome in females, there is a wide variability in Klinefelter syndrome. The description above is the one usually used in textbooks. The mildest cases are probably never diagnosed because their external features are normal. They may even be fertile. The most severe cases have unusual growth patterns, significant behavior or psychiatric problems, and puberty is delayed or absent. Cases of Klinefelter syndrome with more than just one extra X chromosome are more severe. In general, the more chromosomes, the worse the effect.

BOYS TO MEN

Abnormalities in male sexual development can be primary malformations or problems in puberty. Unlike in females, there are normally no internal structures that can harbor "hidden" malformations. Hypospadias, a malformation of the penis, and undescended testicles are common birth defects. They are correctable with surgery, but severe cases may be associated with other problems, particularly of the urinary system. The most common genetic form of male pubertal delay and infertility is 47,XXY (Klinefelter syndrome). This is a kind of testicular failure that usually results in infertility and maturation abnormalities.

Boys at puberty are more likely than girls to have the developing parts of their body exposed to peers. Public restrooms and school showers can be stressful to normal children. When there is an obvious physical problem, that stress is amplified. Parents and schools should be sensitive to these situations.

16 Teenage Angst

When children are young, parents make the decisions. As kids get older, they want and need more input into choices. How much a teenager participates depends upon the person, the situation, and the family. More and more, it is recognized that older kids have the right to be informed and to refuse or assent to a procedure, test, or treatment. They have the right to understand what is going to be done to their bodies and to ask questions.

Likewise, adolescence may be the time to share information about health and disease, normal and abnormal. The last two chapters covered genetic conditions and birth defects that affect sex, sexuality, and reproduction. Other conditions may shorten life spans or increase the risk of health problems. Genetic disease may affect the teen or other family members.

The impulse often is to withhold information—to protect the growing child from bad news. At some point, though, this does not work. Honesty and trust are always the best options. This chapter will not be an in-depth look at adolescent psychology. There is just some advice about watching, listening, and sharing.

RIGHTS AND RESPONSIBILITIES

Going to the doctor starts to change as children grow up. For one thing, children become more aware of where they are. This can be good. It is a chance to meet others facing the same situations: other kids with hearing aids or in wheelchairs or who have seizures. It can be bad if these similar situations are seen as scary or depressing. They start to learn about human biology at school. They are smart enough to look up big words and figure out what they mean.

Teenagers have the right not to be passive participants. They should have an opportunity to ask questions and to get answers. They also can answer questions for themselves instead of deferring to the parent. Depending upon the child, 12 or 13 years is the age at which the physical exam can be done in private—the parent can go to the waiting room. Not only is this respectful, it also gives the patient and doctor a chance to talk.

With some exceptions, physicians legally may not withhold information from the parents. If the teen reports abuse, the authorities must be notified. Otherwise, private moments let the doctor ask the embarrassing questions (sex, drugs, alcohol) with a higher likelihood of getting an honest answer. Also, privacy lets the teenager ask or share things that parental presence inhibits.

Increasingly, medical procedures require the consent of the parents and also the informed assent of the teenager. This includes not only surgery but also the taking of X rays or regular photographs. An intellectually functional 16-year-old should not be ordered to have a surgery or a treatment without explanation. This is also true for participation in research studies. Basically, any medical situation in which there is a legal requirement for patient or guardian informed consent should also include teenager informed assent.

Some persons under age 18 have majority rights. These vary from state to state. Pregnant teens may seek prenatal care without involving their parents. Teenagers may seek psychiatric care or drug treatment on their own. In some states, parenthood confers full majority status regardless of age. In other states, a teenager living apart with personal financial responsibility is an emancipated minor. It is best to know the laws that apply in your area.

With maturing rights come responsibility. You may have been in a doctor's office or hospital that posts patient rights and responsibilities. Teenagers should accept those responsibilities commensurate with the situation—show up, be truthful and complete, follow the treatment provided, etc. Some of these are simple courtesies, such as calling to reschedule an appointment that cannot be kept. Other responsibilities should reflect the growing autonomy of the teen, such as being accountable for monitoring a special diet or taking injections.

HOMOSEXUALITY

As has been discussed, puberty is a time of wild physical and psychological changes. Developing sexuality is a big part of these years. Previous chapters have addressed some of the physical changes. This section will touch briefly on homosexuality, which has gotten quite a bit of scientific attention recently.

In the mid-1990s, a discovery was made that suggested a gene for sexual orientation on the X chromosome. A "gay gene" has not been defined further. There are also some studies showing that male and female humans have somewhat different brain structures and that homosexual men have brains that "look more female." These and other investigations support the idea that homosexuality in men and women has a biologic basis.[1]

Homosexuality is no longer classified as a psychiatric illness. It is considered a normal human variant. There is no genetic test for it. Even if there were, it is unlikely that mainstream genetics would endorse such testing. Testing for sexual orientation would fall under the same umbrella as sex selection. Having one sex or the other, or one sexual orientation or the other, is not a disease.

PERSONAL HEALTH

As mentioned in Chapter 12, children with health problems often figure out that something about them is different. Before they are teenagers they have probably asked questions like: Why do I have to miss school to go to the doctor? Why do I have a scar on my stomach? Why do I have to take medicine? As children ask questions, the best thing to do is give them truthful responses. As the questions become more sophisticated, the answers should match them.

At some point teenagers start asking the "adult" questions. They want the same answers that their parents want. Sometimes this means some research on the family's part. The teen's physician can help, too. This can be a very trying time. It can also be a time to get closer. The problem is something that the teen and the parent have in common. You can attack it together.

Sometimes a teen has inherited a condition but is not yet showing symptoms. At some point he or she will have to know about this. It is not fair to the teen, or later to the adult, to withhold facts until symptoms appear or a major life decision is made. There is no such thing as protecting someone by keeping a secret like this. When the story does finally emerge, a kept secret becomes a betrayal. By the same token, it is unethical to give information in an attempt to control the teen's behavior.

Parents, kids, and their relationships are all different. There is no one best way to help a teenager grow through this time. However, as has been said in previous chapters, communication is always the best place to start. Do not assume. Ask, listen, and keep asking. Talk to your teen about your own concerns—even if they do not seem to be listening, they are hearing you.

Adolescence is typically a time of immortality and invulnerability. Sick or disabled young adults may not have the luxury of believing they are indestructible. This can be frustrating and depressing. Peer pressure is important and fitting in is hard enough without having something that makes one obviously different. On the other hand, kids can adjust amazingly well to chronic illness. They cannot do it on their own, but with support and encouragement they can come to view their differences as uniqueness rather than as curse. Some become role models and poster children, but that is not the goal. The goal is solid self-esteem and a sense that the world is trustworthy.

From the very beginning, children with birth defects or genetic diseases should be treated as normally as possible. Discipline, boundaries, and chores are important. Family rules apply to everybody. Knowing where the lines are drawn gives a framework for decisions. Not only is this good parenting, but it gives the child, and later the teen, a way to succeed. If there are no expectations, no goals, there are no ways to feel accomplishment. It does not matter whether that achievement is tying shoes or getting an A in physics.

FAMILY HEALTH

When a genetic condition runs in the family, an apparently unaffected teenager may still be involved. A teen may have witnessed the effects of disease on another family member. That teen may be the carrier of a recessive mutation or may be nonpenetrant for a dominant one. As with personal health, teenagers will start to question how this other person's illness or disability may affect them.

Whether or not to test an asymptomatic (or presymptomatic) child is an ethical dilemma, even if the child is involved in the decision. Arguments against testing include concerns about future insurance or employment and the possibility that family members will treat the child badly if the test is positive. Regardless of the test results, testing a person before age 18 denies that future adult the right not to know his or her status. This is a subtle point of ethics. Essentially, an adult has a right to remain ignorant of something if he or she chooses. Put another way, an adult has the right not to have information forced upon him or her.

Arguments for testing minors include the right of parents to make medical-testing decisions for their children and to know about potential future health problems. The child's future right not to know may be irrelevant if the family history is clear. Early identification of genetic disease allows for more aggressive educational and financial planning. The information may also be used in family planning.

The American College of Medical Genetics recommends against testing asymptomatic minors to determine if they carry or are predisposed to a genetic disease. Physician practices differ. This author's approach is to advise against testing until the child is old enough to participate meaningfully in the decision to test. The test—positive or negative—does not impact the immediate health of the child. Also, genetic testing technologies are advancing rapidly. Some tests currently take months and cost thousands of dollars. The testing process itself will only get faster and cheaper in the future, so it will be worth the wait.

Occasionally, a parent will request genetic testing in an effort to control a child's sexuality. The reasoning is that a teenager who has a genetic disease can be admonished not to have sex because, if a pregnancy results, the offspring could be affected too. Aside from the fact that this approach probably will not work, there are much better ways to educate teenagers about sexual behavior and sexuality.

LETTING GO

Although it may seem otherwise, children do not suddenly go from infancy to young adult. There are a lot of years between diapers and driving. The difference between the newborn and the teenager is the level of parental control. Growing up is an exercise in taking control or being responsible for oneself. For children with a genetic condition, birth defect, or potential for a genetic disease, there are just more eggs in their basket.

In an ideal situation, the child can start to learn what is going on early. Knowledge and control can increase with age. In some cases, the affected person will never be able to manage alone due to severe mental or physical disability. At the other end of the spectrum are those who are fine until middle age or older. Every person is different—a fact that is also true about people without fancily named conditions.

PART V

Adult Genetic Disease

17 Genetic Conditions That Come on Later

A congenital disease is something present since birth. Technically, all truly genetic conditions are congenital, even those that do not have symptoms until much later. The classic example of these is Huntington disease. Some of these conditions have a peculiar type of genetic change called a repeat mutation. Adult onset and the repeat mutation family of diseases are the subjects of this chapter.

ADULT ONSET

An adult-onset genetic disease is exactly what the name suggests: a condition that does not show up until adulthood. Adulthood is a long time, however, so such a condition may affect 25-year-olds, 80-year-olds, or anyone in between. If symptoms are present since childhood but the diagnosis is not made until later, that is not an adult-onset condition. In an adult-onset condition, the symptoms themselves are delayed or hidden until the grown-up years.

The classic example of an adult-onset genetic disease is Huntington disease. This is a neurologic problem involving the brain. The signs and symptoms are uncontrollable sudden muscle movement, forgetfulness, clumsiness, and lack of coordination. Huntington disease also affects cognitive ability and mood. As the disease progresses, affected persons lose the ability to walk, speak, or swallow. Death is from choking, infection, or heart failure. Symptoms of Huntington disease usually start in the thirties and forties, although the youngest reported patient was two years old. It affects males and females equally and is inherited in a dominant fashion (see Chapter 6).

We all accept that we will have health problems of some sort as we get older. There are two aspects of adult-onset genetic disease that are particularly troublesome. The first is that they impair health both more severely and earlier than expected. Everyone expects to have health problems associated with aging in their seventies and later, but not in their forties. The second is that the condition may be unknowingly passed to children. The symptoms often do not show up until after the reproductive years. A person ignorant of their genetic status will have had children by the time the diagnosis is made. Adult-onset genetic diseases are most commonly dominant. This means that an affected person has a 50% chance of passing the mutated gene to each of his or her children.

Genetic disease is usually thought of as something that shows up in childhood. A prospective parent has a sibling or nephew or aunt who was born with a problem. It is easy to correlate: birth or infant problems in the family make it prudent to investigate before a pregnancy. Health problems in a 70-year-old, or even a 50-year-old, relative are not considered risky for a newborn. It is easy to make the connection once the disease is diagnosed, but that may be after the birth of many children.

In strict evolutionary terms, adult-onset genetic diseases stay in the population because affected persons live long enough to reproduce. The chance of passing the mutation to a child is high enough that, adding everyone together, each generation is as affected as the one before it. Diseases that are lethal before reproductive age, or that impair fertility, tend to become rare. They do not go away completely because new mutations happen all the time.

REPEAT MUTATION

There is a rather old concept in medical diagnosis called anticipation. If a parent or other family member was diagnosed with a genetic condition in adulthood, subsequent children were diagnosed at younger ages. This was thought to be an artifact. The doctor was more alert and knew what to look for, so was finding the symptoms earlier in the children. The doctor was *anticipating* the appearance of disease in the child. It turns out that, in some hereditary diseases, the children really are more severely affected than the parents. So, the clinical definition of anticipation has changed, but it is still present.

Anticipation has a molecular definition as well, and it applies to a particular type of genetic change called a repeat mutation. As explained in Chapter 5, genes and DNA are made up of four bases: A, C, G, and T. The order of the bases determines the role of the gene. In some genes there are strings of bases that repeat themselves. These can be pairs (**CG**CG**CG**CG**CG**), triplets (**CGG**CGG**CGG**CGG**CGG**), or larger. It is normal to have some number of repeats.

Sometimes the number of repeats in the string increases. This usually happens during recombination — when the paired chromosomes trade pieces before making eggs and sperm. If the repeat gets significantly larger, if it expands, then the gene becomes unstable. The repeat expansion is a mutation that causes disease.

Huntington disease is a triplet repeat expansion disease. The gene is called HD and is located at the upper tip of chromosome 4. The protein is called Huntingtin. The disease is caused by a triplet repeat: CAG **CAG**CAG. Having 10 to 26 triplets is normal. If there are 36 or more repeats, a full expansion, Huntington disease happens. People with repeats numbering 27 to 35 triplets will probably not have symptoms but are at risk for having children with the full expansion. This is called having a premutation. The number of repeats in a full expansion mutation is indirectly correlated with the onset of disease — the more repeats, the younger the symptoms appear.

Another common triplet repeat expansion disease is Fragile X syndrome. This is a mental retardation syndrome that affects mostly males. The gene is called FMR1 (Fragile X Mental Retardation gene 1) and is located at Xq27.3, near the bottom end of the X chromosome. The protein is called FMRP (Fragile X Mental Retardation Protein). Fragile X is an X-linked condition, so how severely a person is affected depends on both the size of the repeat expansion and the sex of the patient. Females are not as severely affected as males.

Fragile X disease got its name because of the way the X chromosome can look under the microscope. When the cells are grown in a nutrient that lacks folic acid — an important B vitamin — the end of the X chromosome looks like it is broken off, hence "Fragile." It was noticed that this happens in the cells of mentally retarded males who have a particular set of features and symptoms. The similarity of the patients, and the repeated finding of the "Fragile" X, led to the disease discovery.

In Fragile X the normal number of repeats is 5 to 44. The range from 45 repeats to 54 is a gray zone. Persons with this size repeat do not have the disease, but there is a significant risk that the repeat will expand in future generations. The premutation range for Fragile X is 55 to 200 repeats. Repeat sizes over 200 to 230 cause disease. Repeat sizes can be huge — too big to measure with conventional technology. As the repeat size grows, the degree of mental retardation increases.

The known triplet repeat expansion diseases are degenerative brain and nerve conditions. In addition to Huntington disease and Fragile X there is also myotonic dystrophy, Friedreich ataxia, spinal and bulbar muscular atrophy, and others. There are about 20 discovered to date. They are all autosomal dominant except for Fragile X, which is X-linked.

For a while Fragile X appeared to be different from the others because of inheritance and because it was not degenerative. It is now known that males with premutations — repeats sized 55 to 200 — develop an adult-onset condition called Fragile X-Associated Tremor/Ataxia Syndrome (FXTAS). This can also affect female premutation carriers, although it is usually milder in them.

One other unusual thing about this set of diseases is that it matters whether it is passed on from the mother or the father. In some of them, the premutation will become a full expansion only if inherited from the parent of a particular sex. Huntington disease worsens as it passes through men. Fragile X and myotonic dystrophy get worse if they come from the mother. The reason for this is not yet known.

GENETIC TESTING

In the early days of gene discovery, the general location of the HD gene was established even though the gene itself was not known. Predictive or diagnostic testing could be done through a process called linkage analysis. This test was informative — it gave a definitive positive or negative answer — about 96% of the time. Four percent of the time the test was uninformative. Thus, patients would receive one of three answers: you inherited the mutation; you did not inherit the mutation; or the test was not useful. Now that the HD gene is known and the triplet repeat mutation is characterized, it is possible in 99+% of patients to give a definitive answer right down to the number of repeats that a person has.

It can be devastating to get the diagnosis of a future disease. Studying people who had the old linkage test for Huntington disease showed that different people were affected by different stress. Persons who had a positive test, a diagnosis of Huntington, had high levels of stress or anxiety immediately, but it eventually diminished to normal. Persons with a negative test generally felt relief but could experience "survivor guilt" because they were healthy while siblings were not. This kind of stress is individual and family dependent. Persons with the uninformative test result had no stress initially, but then it built up over time. The conclusion from this is that having no answer is worse over the long term than having bad news.

When the Huntington disease and other adult-onset disease genes were found, geneticists thought that there would be many people requesting the tests. It was assumed that anyone with a positive family history would want to know their own genotype. This has turned out not to be true. For a variety of reasons, people are choosing not to be tested.

ALL PREDICTIONS ARE LIMITED

There is a protocol in place for persons who wish to be tested for Huntington disease. It involves pretest and posttest counseling and the involvement of family members. This is the only genetic condition for which such a system exists. There is some disagreement among geneticists about using a process like this for one disease and not for others.

It is often difficult for doctors or other health care providers to predict what will cause psychological stress. There is one story told of a man with a family history of Huntington disease. He had a 50:50 chance of having inherited the mutation. For some reason, he was convinced that he had, indeed, inherited the disease and that he would die by the time he was 50. He lived a very full life every day, played hard, did not marry or have children, and did not save for his old age. When he finally was tested he found out that his HD genes were both normal. He was not affected.

18 Genetics of Common Adult Diseases

In Chapter 3 we discussed the concept of multifactorial diseases. These are what they sound like: conditions caused by many different factors. Some of these factors are genetic and some are not. As we live our lives, we are exposed to more and more of the nongenetic factors. Some of the factors are individually controllable: one can choose to smoke or not. Other factors may be controllable on a neighborhood or society level, such as clean indoor air laws or forcing a polluting factory to shut down. Some exposures are beyond our ability to control, such as cosmic radiation.

The unknown is what combination of factors matters. The bag of marbles example in Figure 3.2 works whether the condition is a cleft lip or Alzheimer disease. As with birth defects, the adult multifactorial diseases are an area of active research. There is one nuance of semantics: while the term "multifactorial" is technically correct for all diseases with some genetic component, it is often used only to apply to birth defects. Adult diseases such as Alzheimer, Parkinson, and coronary artery disease are referred to as "common adult diseases."

This chapter uses Alzheimer disease and breast cancer to demonstrate the complex nature of common adult disease genetics. These are both good examples of why multifactorial diseases are so difficult to predict and treat. In addition, the discussion of breast cancer can be an overview for our current understanding of cancer pathogenesis.

ALZHEIMER DISEASE

Alzheimer disease (AD) is a degenerative disease of the brain that is associated with loss of brain cells. The cardinal feature of AD is dementia, which is a decline in thinking skills: loss of memory, problems in reasoning, disorientation, and so on. People with dementia can also have changes in their behavior and psychoses such as delusions and hallucinations. AD overlaps with other brain diseases, and specific diagnosis based on symptoms alone can be difficult or delayed. As more research is done, it may be found that what we now call Alzheimer disease is, in fact, a number of different conditions with similar signs and symptoms.[1]

About 15–25% of the time, Alzheimer disease is inherited in an autosomal dominant fashion. In these families an affected person has a 50:50 chance of having an affected child. Since this is an adult-onset condition, it may be more reasonably thought of from the offspring point of view: when a parent is diagnosed with AD, the child has a 50:50 chance of also developing it. Symptoms of familial Alzheimer disease also tend to appear at younger ages. There is a specific type of familial Alzheimer that is called "early-onset familial Alzheimer disease." It accounts for less than 2% of all AD cases, and symptoms consistently occur earlier than 65 years of age.

In the other 75% of families, AD is multifactorial. When one person is diagnosed, the risk to first-degree relatives (parents, children, and siblings) is 10–50% that they will also be affected. The risk increases with age. It is also recognized that persons with trisomy 21 (Down syndrome) are at very high risk of developing AD, particularly at an earlier age. This is because of the trisomy 21 rather than a high family risk. Persons with trisomy 21 account for less than 1% of all AD patients.

There are two known biochemical brain abnormalities associated with AD: fibrillary proteins (Tau proteins) in the brain nerve cells and amyloid b-peptide (amyloid plaques) in the extracellular spaces. Genes that code for both of these proteins are known. There is also an association between AD and a protein called Apolipoprotein E.

The amyloid precursor protein gene (APP) is located on chromosome 21. This may account for the increased risk of AD in persons with trisomy 21. The normal function of the gene is not known at this time. There are multiple different mutations in the gene that are thought to be pathogenic (disease causing). Some mutations cause familial AD. Other mutations cause regular late-onset AD. One mutation is associated with schizophrenia. The effect of these mutations is not completely clear, but it is thought that they lead to overproduction of the protein, which, in turn, disrupts the function of the cell. Normal production of the APP is dependent upon two other proteins, Presenilin 1 and 2. Mutations in the genes for these proteins are also recognized to cause early-onset AD.

One of the other proteins in an amyloid plaque is Apolipoprotein E. Abnormalities in the gene for this protein, located on chromosome 19, cause late-onset AD. Briefly, there are three known alleles (versions) of the *APOE* gene designated *e2*, *e3*, and *e4*. The most common is *e3*. In a given person there may be any of six possible pairs of these alleles: *e2e2*, *e2e3*, *e2e4*, *e3e3*, *e3e4*, or *e4e4*. There is an increased chance that a person with AD will have *e4*. If both *APOE* alleles are *e4*, and the person gets AD, then he or she will develop the symptoms earlier. On the other hand, the *e2* allele is protective. In the presence of even one *e2* allele, the overall risk of AD is slightly lower, and if it does occur, symptoms will occur later. Unfortunately, these associations only work in persons of European descent.

Apolipoprotein E has received coverage in general medical literature because it is part of a test for heart disease risk. In the process of doing tests to evaluate for coronary artery disease, cardiologists may test Apolipoprotein E. An ethical dilemma arose when it became clear that the test in some patients would show more than just information about heart disease. The test might also show an increased risk for AD. Cardiologists were not prepared to counsel patients about a disease outside their field of medicine. When this test is done now, it is typical for a patient to be advised up-front that the result may indicate health risks other than, or in addition to, the problem for which the test is being sent.

The Tau protein is the other major protein associated with Alzheimer disease. It has a known function. It promotes microtubule formation and stabilization. Microtubules are scaffold structures in the cell that support cell shape and facilitate the movement of some structures around the inside of the cell. There are a number of different Tau proteins all coded for by the same gene. Which protein is produced depends upon how the gene, located on chromosome 17, is processed. Mutations in or dysfunction of Tau leads to dysfunction of the microtubules, which disrupts the cell.

There are diseases caused by just an abnormality in the Tau protein, which suggests that the dementia in AD is related to the Tau protein and not the amyloid plaque. The presenilins, APP, and Tau may be different steps in a single metabolic process. The Apolipoprotein E would then contribute to the disease but not be a primary causative agent.

AD is a great example of a multifactorial genetic condition. As demonstrated, there are multiple known genes involved. Each gene has many possible disease-causing mutations. In addition, there is at least one protein that contributes, even if it does not cause the condition. Environmentally, there are possible associations between head trauma and nicotine use and the risk for Alzheimer disease. This complexity makes it difficult to have a single clear diagnosis or treatment and makes risk assessment imprecise. As many as 1 person in 10 will have some form of memory or intellectual impairment when they are past 70 years of age. About half of these have AD. This is a very large number of people to have one condition, but there are still many other brain diseases that need to be considered.

BREAST CANCER

Breast cancer, as with most cancers, is not a single disease. Not only are there multiple different types of breast cancer, the causes for each are numerous. Only a small percentage are clearly genetic in origin. Overall, the risk for breast cancer increases with age, and it is much more common in, but not exclusive to, females. Other factors that play a role are smoking, hormone use, age of menarche, age of menopause, number of children, presence of benign breast disease, and exposure to high levels of radiation.

All cancer is genetic in that it is caused by a change in DNA. However, it is not all heritable. As was discussed in Chapter 2, genetic, familial, and heritable are three different concepts. They overlap, but they are not all true all the time. The vast majority of breast cancer is not inherited—it is sporadic. That is why all women are at risk. Only about 15–20% of breast cancer happens in women who have a positive family history for the disease. Even in some of those cases, the disease is not caused by a single, easily identified gene.

As with any multifactorial disease, a woman (or man) is at increased risk for breast cancer if there are other members of the family affected. The more unusual or severe the case in the affected person, the higher the risk to family members. For example, if the affected person is male or is under 45, the risk to family members is greater than if the patient is female and over 90.

There are two known breast cancer susceptibility genes: *BRCA1* and *BRCA2*. Although these two genes together account for only about 5% of breast cancer, there is high penetrance in families with inherited mutations. Inherited breast cancers due to one of these genes have more severe characteristics than multifactorial cancers. They tend to manifest at younger ages, be bilateral, and be associated with tumors in other organs.

Women with a mutation in one of these genes have an almost 100% risk of developing breast and/or ovarian cancer by age 85.

The *BRCA1* gene is located on chromosome 17 and may account for 20–30% of the inherited breast cancers (approximately 1.25% of all breast cancers). Women with a mutation in this gene also have an increased risk of ovarian cancer. *BRCA2* is the other known breast cancer susceptibility gene and is on chromosome 13. It is thought to account for 10–20% of all inherited breast cancers (approximately 1% of all breast cancers). There is some increased risk of ovarian cancer, but not as high as with *BRCA1* mutations. There is a higher risk to men when the gene mutation in the family involves *BRCA2*.

In families with *BRCA1* or *BRCA2* mutations, breast cancer is inherited in an autosomal dominant fashion. This means that, looking at the pedigree, an affected person has a 50:50 chance of having an affected child. However, there are two major steps to the development of cancer, so what is really inherited is not the cancer but a risk of, or susceptibility to, cancer. (It is important to remember that everyone has the genes *BRCA1* and *BRCA2*. The names come from the disease they cause when abnormal, but they both have a normal function that is important. They only contribute to cancer when there is a mutation.)

There are two copies, two alleles, for every gene. In a heritable cancer, the parent passes on a mutated allele, but the child's other allele, inherited from the other parent, is normal. As long as the normal allele is functioning, there is no cancer. The cancer starts when a mutation happens in the normal allele in the susceptible part of the body. Changes in DNA happen all the time as cells grow and divide. Usually the cellular repair machinery takes care of the problem. Occasionally it does not. When a change happens in a cancer gene that has no normal partner and the DNA repair mechanisms do not catch it, the cancer starts.

This is called Knudson's two-hit hypothesis of cancer. Hit number 1 is the inheritance of a mutated allele in a cancer susceptibility gene. Hit number 2 is the development of a mutation in the normal allele. This holds true for all the heritable cancers. This gets tricky because the mutation itself is recessive: as long as the normal allele is functioning, the disease does not manifest. However, the susceptibility to the cancer is dominant: it is passed from parent to child with a 50% risk.

Even when there is a breast cancer gene mutation in a family, it is still impossible to be completely precise about the risk of developing cancer. The numbers quoted above start with women who already have the disease: of all women with cancer, *x* have a mutation. That is easy because that is a simple head count. It is more difficult to determine whether a woman with the mutation will develop cancer. There is no way to know all of the women with the mutation, so it will never be possible to say: of all women with the mutation, x will have cancer. Some women will not develop cancer in their lifetimes, so they would not be counted or countable.

The reader will also note that *BRCA1* and *BRCA2* together are thought to account for only 30–50% of all inherited cancers (approximately 5% of all breast cancer). This means that some families with clearly inherited breast cancer must have a mutation in a different gene. There are a few known cancer syndromes that have breast cancer as a feature, and there are other single genes, such as the estrogen receptor gene, that may be involved in breast cancer specifically.

NO RISK IS 100%

As we age our risk of having a common age-related disease increases. With growing knowledge it may become possible to decrease our risk of various conditions such as Alzheimer disease and cancer. Right now, changes in diet and lifestyle are the most commonly recommended ways to maximize future health. But in the developed world, there are also more people living to the age of 100 in reasonable health. These people, because of good living or genetics or luck, have avoided the risks of many potential conditions.

19 Knowledge Is Power

This book has discussed birth defects and genetic disease from conception through adulthood. It has also touched on some related topics that are important to families dealing with these diseases. Each section has had a chapter about the ethical, legal, or psychological issues that can arise at each stage of life or rite of passage. In discussion about adult diseases, and a finish to the book, this chapter covers some end-of-life matters. These things are important to everyone, not just people with genetic diseases or birth defects. As presented, they apply specifically to persons age 18 and over living in the United States. Applications in other countries may vary.

In adult life in the United States, there are three major medically related legal issues: legal guardianship, living wills, and durable power of attorney for health care (DPAHC). The laws that govern these processes vary from state to state. Specific questions about how these apply to you or your family should be addressed to your doctor, a social worker, or an attorney.

Since this chapter deals with legal issues, some definitions are necessary. A person 18 years of age or older is competent by default. Only a judge can declare that a legal adult is incompetent and take away that person's right to make financial, living, and medical decisions. If someone is declared incompetent, that person is assigned a legal guardian, which is discussed below.

A person can be legally competent but lack the capacity to make medical decisions for himself or herself. This is not a legal finding. It can

Table 19.1   Four Questions to Assess the Capacity to Make Medical Decisions
(The patient is having seizures. The doctor is recommending an EEG—a test
that measures brain electricity. It is done by putting sensors against the scalp.
There are no needles. Nothing is put into the skin.)

	Question	Acceptable Answer	Unacceptable Answer
1	What is your diagnosis?	Seizures	Muscle spasms
2	What is your doctor recommending?	An EEG test	He wants to put wires into my brain
3	What will happen if you accept/refuse this treatment?	The test should show the seizures and what part of the brain is involved	If I refuse, the nurses will poison me
4	Why are you accepting/refusing this treatment	I want the doctor to learn as much as possible to help me	I'm refusing because the doctor will use the EEG to control my thoughts

be determined by any physician. Table 19.1 shows four questions that
can be used to determine capacity to make medical decisions. Examples
of acceptable and unacceptable answers are given. Basically, the patient
must understand what is wrong, the suggested treatment, and the risks
and benefits of the treatment. The patient must also have a logical or reasonable reason for accepting or rejecting a particular treatment.

Capacity may be impaired long term, as in mental retardation, or
temporarily, as in a concussion because of a car accident. When an otherwise competent adult lacks the capacity to make medical decisions, the
decision will fall to the closest available next of kin. By default, this is
usually a spouse, parent, or adult child. This designation varies by state
and can be overridden by patient wishes. This representative person is
called the surrogate decision maker. The surrogate should make medical
care decisions based upon what the patient's wishes would be and what
is in the best interest of the patient. The surrogate's responsibility ends
when the patient regains the capacity to make decisions or is declared
incompetent and assigned a legal guardian.

LEGAL GUARDIANSHIP

Parents are the legal guardians of children under age 18. At 18, individuals become autonomous or competent. They are legally allowed to
make all decisions for themselves. By default, all persons are presumed
to be capable of managing their own affairs. Mental retardation, mental
illness, or physical disability does not make someone incompetent. Persons so affected have the same rights as unaffected persons.

Sometimes an adult is not capable of making medical decisions and of
managing other business. This may be true because of mental retardation,

dementia, severe injury, or other illness. In these cases, it is best for the person to have a legal guardian who can help handle things. Guardians also help protect the assisted adult from being mistreated. The legal guardian has, essentially, the same obligation as a parent.

Guardians are assigned by the court system. Often, a legal guardian is a relative, but there are no restrictions on who can be someone's legal guardian. As in parenting, the responsibility of the guardian varies with the functioning of the ward. A patient in a coma requires someone to make all decisions. An adult with trisomy 21 who lives in a group home and holds a job needs a different level of guardian involvement.

DURABLE POWER OF ATTORNEY FOR HEALTH CARE

The durable power of attorney for health care (DPAHC) has a bulky name. It is important to know that the DPAHC is separate from a durable power of attorney that gives someone power over financial affairs. The DPAHC is limited to medical decisions. It designates who may be the surrogate decision maker for someone. This designation overrides state law that assigns a surrogate. The person named in the DPAHC should be someone who can express the wishes of the patient, not his or her own wishes.

The DPAHC is a legal document that is executed while a person (future patient) is mentally functional. It can be done at any time and is generally recommended for all adults. The specific wording may vary among states. In general, a competent adult uses the DPAHC to appoint a first-choice and a second-choice surrogate. The surrogate indicated by a DPAHC supersedes anyone else who may otherwise have legal rights. For example, the DPAHC may assign surrogate decision making to a sibling in a state where a spouse would be the default.

The DPAHC may also indicate what sort of decisions the surrogate can make. A surrogate may be granted the right to make decisions about surgery or kidney dialysis but not decisions about starting or withdrawing a breathing machine. A DPAHC is usually used in conjunction with a living will, although the living will takes precedence. Again, the specific rights of a surrogate may be different in your state.

LIVING WILL

A living will, or directive to physicians, is a document that indicates how persons want to be treated at the end of life when they are no longer able to speak for themselves. It only becomes effective when the patient permanently lacks decision-making capacity, there are no treatment options, and the caregivers agree that further medical procedures would be futile. As defined in Chapter 12, medical futility is the point at which no treatment will cure or improve the situation. A living will would not become effective, for example, for someone undergoing surgery or for an unconscious patient who is expected to recover. A living will is never in effect as long as the patient is able to state wishes directly.

If someone has a living will, then it is clear to both doctors and family members what that individual wants. It does not imply a particular decision. A patient may indicate in the living will that they wish everything done for as long as possible. More commonly, though, people use living wills to say that they do not wish to have their bodies kept alive by machines if they would otherwise die.

A living will may have clauses that separately discuss the use of breathing machines, kidney dialysis, antibiotics, cardiopulmonary resuscitation (CPR), and certain medications. It can be as detailed or as general as a person wishes. There is no right or wrong way to fill in a living will. Its only function is to make sure that an individual's wishes are known.

Living wills are best completed by all healthy adults. They can be altered or adjusted over time, just like wills that dispose of material things. Decisions that seem right at age 30 may not be right at age 80. One is never too young to have a living will because it is impossible to predict when it may be needed. Once it is executed, make multiple copies. The more people who know about it, the greater chance that it will be followed. In addition to having one easily available, a copy can go to the patient's primary doctor, lawyer, a family member, and someone at the patient's place of worship.

At least as important as the paper itself is the discussion about it. As with making the decision to be an organ donor, the decision is irrelevant if it is a secret. Going through the process of making a living will means talking to your doctor, your family, and maybe your lawyer. Talking gets your feelings out in the open. Some people are not comfortable thinking about their own mortality. However, living wills are not about death. They are about having some control over the end of life.

THE LAST WORD

Genetics is a complex science. Genetic changes can enhance, damage, or end life. Any single change may be rare, but added together the changes affect all of us. A change in genetics may cause problems at any time from conception to old age. This book has been an overview. For each life stage there has been a discussion of the problems that may arise and some of the things about which to be aware.

Genetics is a growing science. Almost every aspect of human biology eventually comes back to genetics. In 1983 the AIDS virus was identified by describing how it looked under a microscope. Twenty years later the SARS virus was identified by sequencing its genome. Geneticists used to joke that even the chance that someone gets the flu is genetic. While this book was being written, the first solid proof of the relationship between genetics and susceptibility to infection was published.

Genetics is a fascinating science. It's like learning the secret of a magic trick. It's a peek inside Mother Nature's bag of tricks. Sometimes what we see just raises more questions. Other times it's like suddenly finding the instruction manual. And it's never dull.

Appendices

Appendix A:
Models of Genetic Risk

There are two models used to discuss the interpersonal variation in disease risk: the Basic Model and the Threshold Model. In some conditions one model is more useful than the other, although both can be used at some level for anything.

THE BASIC MODEL

The Basic Model is useful when discussing differences that manifest somehow in everyone, such as height. A person's final height is determined by genes and nutrition. As a simple example, assume that height is determined by one gene and one nutrient. The gene has two alleles that can come in three possible combinations: TT, Tt, and tt. Allele T makes people tall and allele t makes people short. So, persons inheriting TT are tall, those with tt are short, and those with Tt are in between. (Detailed discussion of genes and alleles can be found in Chapter 5.) In addition, there is a nutrient we'll call Z. The more of Z that a child eats, the taller that child will grow—within the limits of his or her genetics. If no Z is eaten, the height is determined by genetics alone. Figure A.1 shows the various combinations that result.

Obviously, human height is not determined by just one gene and one nutrient and people do not grow to just a few height cutoff points. If more genes or nutrients are added to the graph in Figure A.1, it would start to look like the graph in Figure A.2. Finally, with the addition of sufficient factors, the bar graph would smooth out to a curve, which more accurately represents the real variation in human height.

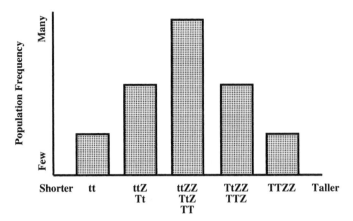

Figure A.1   The Basic Model of multifactorial inheritance. Example: height— various combinations of gene and nutrients lead to different heights. There is only one combination at each end of the spectrum, so fewer people are included in that part of the graph. The most common height, that in the middle of the spectrum, is caused by three possible combinations.

The Basic Model can be used to demonstrate or estimate disease risk: the statistical likelihood that someone will be affected with a disease. Overall risk is distributed so that there are a few people with very low risk, a few people with very high risk, and everyone else in between. Most people have average risk. This distribution is represented by a bell-shaped curve, also called a Gaussian curve or a normal distribution curve. Figure A.2 is a bar graph demonstrating the increasing steps of risk and the percentage of the population included in each risk level. The superimposed smooth curve is the normal distribution that results when enough points are added to the equation.

In the Basic Model, everyone has some degree of risk. The risk is never zero, although it is very low for some people. The risk is never 100% until an actual diagnosis is made. Also, risk of disease changes over time, since age and exposure are important. Getting older means that genes are at higher risk of accumulating mutations and there has been longer exposure to detrimental things such as air pollution.

Using the bag of marbles analogy in the Basic Model would mean that everyone has a bag with some marbles in it and all bags are at risk of breaking. Some people have bags with just a few marbles, so the risk of breakage is low (but not impossible). Other people's bags have many marbles, so the risk is high (although not guaranteed). Most people fall somewhere in the middle, in the normal distribution.

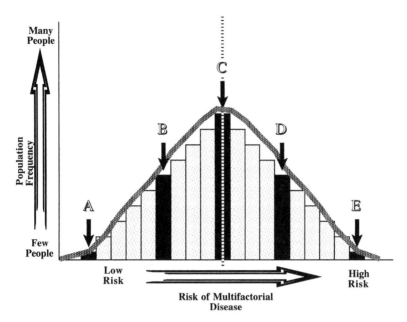

Figure A.2   Normal distribution of multifactorial disease risk. The horizontal axis measures risk from low to high. The vertical axis measures the number of people involved. Each column represents the number of people whose risk is that particular amount. The dotted vertical line marks the division of the population. Half of the population is above (to the right) of the line and has more than average risk. Half the population is below (to the left) of the line and has less than average risk. Letters A to E indicate specific points along the curve as examples. The gray line is the normal distribution curve obtained when enough data are added to the calculation. A = very low risk, very few people; B = moderately low risk, many people; C = average risk, very many people; D = moderately high risk, many people; E = very high risk, very few people.

In this model, it is not possible to compare two different conditions with each other and maintain the Gaussian curve. If a condition has a different risk than normal distribution, the shape of the graph changes. The Basic Model is useful only when discussing a single entity in a large population.

THE THRESHOLD MODEL

The other model is the Threshold Model. It uses the same normal distribution curve as the Basic Model but offers a different interpretation. The Threshold Model is useful for conditions or disease risk that are either present or not, such as the birth defect pyloric stenosis—a blockage between the stomach and the small intestine. The idea here is that there is no risk at all until a particular degree of liability is reached. Below that threshold the disease or condition does not occur, regardless of the presence of liability factors. Figure A.3 describes this idea.

Going back to the bag of marbles, the Threshold Model says that all bags are intact up to a certain point. After that point is reached, all bags break. There is no risk of breakage at all when there are just a few marbles or even an average number of marbles.

In this model it is possible to compare different conditions. These are no absolute numbers, as those would not mean anything and would be impossible to calculate. Rather, the threshold can be manipulated on the graph to compare two multifactorial conditions with each other. The threshold is lowered by moving the cutoff point to the left and raised by moving it to the right.

Some multifactorial birth defects affect the two sexes differently. Cleft lip is more common in males than in females. All other things being equal—family history, birth order, maternal nutrition, and so on—males are at a higher risk of being born with a cleft lip than females. This is an observed phenomenon. Using the Threshold Model to demonstrate this idea yields Figure A.4. Note that the threshold is at a different point in the graph for each of the two sexes.

These models are used as a way to discuss various conditions and risks. They are based upon observations. The flow of information is as

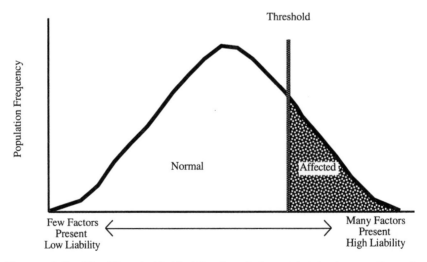

Figure A.3 The Threshold Model of multifactorial inheritance. Example: pyloric stenosis.

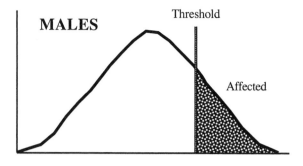

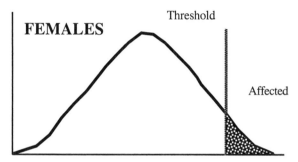

Figure A.4   Male versus female cleft lip risk demonstrated by the Threshold Model.

follows: (1) observation of phenomenon; (2) construction of the measurement/prediction model; (3) use of the model for prediction in other phenomena. It should be remembered that the models are based upon things that manifest in certain ways. A given model may not be useful when the situation is different from the one used to construct the model.

Appendix B:
Influences on Dominant
Genetic Conditions

Dominant genetic conditions are inherited in an all-or-none fashion: either the mutation is there or it is not. However, manifestation of these conditions varies, even within a family. There are three phenomena that are used to describe the variable presentation of dominant diseases — penetrance, expressivity, and anticipation.

PENETRANCE

With some dominant conditions it is possible to be heterozygous for the mutant allele but not show the condition. Such a person is said to be "nonpenetrant" for the disease or the mutation. These people are identified most commonly by having both an affected parent and an affected child. The nonpenetrant person must have the mutation, inherited from his or her own parent and then passed to the next generation. Figure B.1 is the pedigree of such a family. The person indicated by the arrow is nonpenetrant. She has to have the mutation because both her father and son have it, but she does not show any features. Genetic testing can confirm in some cases that the mutation is present but not manifesting.

The *penetrance* of a dominant condition is a ratio or a percentage. In essence, it is the number of people with the phenotype (manifesting the disease) compared with the number of people with the genotype (having the mutation). It is discussed scientifically as a percentage:

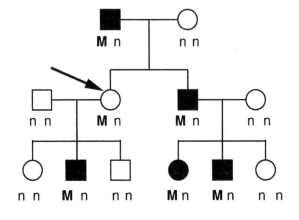

M = Mutant Allele   n = Normal Allele

Figure B.1 Variable penetrance of a dominant genetic condition. The woman indicated by the arrow has the mutated gene but does not manifest the condition. She is nonpenetrant for the condition. The family member with the filled symbol is both heterozygous and penetrant.

$$\frac{\text{Number of people with phenotype}}{\text{Number of people with genotype}} = \text{Percent penetrance.}$$

Penetrance does not define how severely someone is affected. It is only a measure of whether any features of the condition are present. Please note that the correct term is "penetrance," not "penetration."

A simple analogy is a classroom of students all wearing different colors. All the students wearing blue are penetrant for the "blue shirt allele." A single student who is wearing red, but who owns a blue shirt, is nonpenetrant.

EXPRESSIVITY

Expressivity is the range of phenotypes that may be manifested by a particular genotype. It helps define the variable severity of a dominant condition. Using the student analogy above, of all those wearing blue shirts, some have on stripes, some solids, some prints or plaids. They are all penetrant for the "blue shirt allele," but they all express it differently.

Expressivity is a subjective measure based upon the physical exam of a particular patient. A patient may have low or high expressivity as

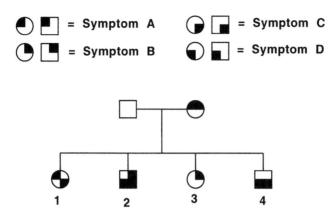

Figure B.2 Variable expressivity. Each affected family member has a different constellation of features, although they all have the same condition. The mother has symptoms A and B. Daughter 1 has symptoms A and C. Son 2 is the most affected and has symptoms A, B, and C. Daughter 3 is the least affected and has only symptom B.

assessed against the baseline for a disease. There is no strict mathematical formula, but it may be thought of as

$$\frac{\text{Phenotype in a particular individual}}{\text{Most severe phenotype for the condition}} = \text{Expressivity}.$$

Figure B.2 is a pedigree showing variable expressivity. Different sections of the symbols are filled in to indicate the presence of different phenotypic features, different symptoms of the condition. This is a complicated but very informative way to draw a family pedigree. Even without knowing the specific symptoms, it is easy to see that no two patterns are the same. Basic information about pedigree symbols can be found in Chapter 2.

ANTICIPATION

Sometimes, when a particular disease runs in a family, children are diagnosed at a young age. It is thought that doctors anticipate the presence of disease and find symptoms earlier than they would otherwise. This is good use of the family history and is still true in many conditions. This is called clinical anticipation.

There is a subset of genetic diseases that really do get worse as they pass through the generations. They are caused by a particular type of mutation called a repeat mutation. The gene is disrupted by a repeating pattern of bases. The more the bases repeat, the worse the disruption to the gene and the more serious the disease. This is called molecular anticipation. In younger generations the symptoms may be more severe—worse mental retardation, worse neurologic disease—or the symptoms may start at a younger age. Chapter 17 discusses this subset of conditions in detail.

Notes

I WHAT IS A GENETICS DOCTOR?

1. More information about training and certification in genetics can be found on the American Board of Medical Genetics website at http://www.abmg.org/.

2 PRIMER ON FAMILY HISTORY

1. Hemophilia and its precise genetic transmission are described in the Talmud (Yebamot 64b).

2. In medical jargon, the term "abortion" means an interruption of pregnancy prior to 20 weeks. It applies both to miscarriages—spontaneous abortions—and elective terminations.

3. National Center for Health Statistics, Centers for Disease Control and Prevention, Atlanta, GA, 2001. World Wide Web URL: http://www.cdc.gov/nchs/.

3 WHO IS AFFECTED BY GENETIC DISEASE?

1. http://www.gwu.edu/~cms/aviation/track_i/barnett.htm.

2. Professor Arnold Barnett, as quoted in *The Oregonian*, February 6, 2000.

4 DNA, CHROMOSOMES, AND GENES

1. Dr. Francis Crick, who described the structure of DNA with Dr. James Watson, died on July 28, 2004, just as this book was being submitted.

2. There are variations on the basic shape of DNA. For example, there is a form of DNA that turns backwards called Z-DNA. Discussion of these variations is beyond the scope of this book, but there are good explanations in any formal genetics textbook.

3. Well, he may have fudged a little.

4. The number after the "q" is read "two, one" rather than "twenty-one." What is missing is band 2, subband 1. There is no band 21. Chromosomes are numbered one to twenty-two. All numbers indicating bands in karyotypes are read as individual numbers one to nine. For example, 22q11.2 is not "twenty-two-q-eleven-point-two"; it is "twenty-two-q-one-one-point-two."

5   FOREWARNED AND FOREARMED

1. Henshaw SK. Unintended pregnancy in the United States. Fam Plann Perspect. 1998;30(1):24–29,46.

2. Floyd RL, Decouflé P, Hungerford DW. Alcohol use prior to pregnancy recognition. Am J Prev Med. 1999;17(2):101–107.

3. Andres RL, Day MC. Perinatal complications associated with maternal tobacco use. Semin Neonatol. 2000;5(3):231–241.

4. Hultman CM, Sparen P, Cnattingius S. Perinatal risk factors for infantile autism. Epidemiology. 2002;13(4):417–423.

6   WHEN GENETIC DISEASE RUNS IN A FAMILY

1. There is a closed Orthodox Jewish community in New York that has successfully eliminated some common recessive diseases in its children by controlling who may marry whom.

7   HIDDEN GENETIC RISKS

1. This is commonly used industry jargon. It is generally not considered offensive.

2. The idea behind Haldane's method is based upon the idea that each gene has a mutation rate that is calculable and that male and female mutation rates differ. A detailed explanation can be found in Vogel and Motulsky's *Human Genetics*. Springer: New York; 1997:395.

9   WHAT IF A TEST IS POSITIVE?

1. The Alan Guttmacher Institute, Facts in brief: Induced abortion, http://www.agiusa.org/pubs/fb_induced_abortion.html; and Gold RB. *Abortion and*

Women's Health: A Turning Point for America? New York: The Alan Guttmacher Institute; 1990.

2. I use the term "offering" rather than "giving up" very specifically. Releasing a child for adoption is a gift—both to the child and to the new family. It is a profoundly altruistic thing to do.

10   ABNORMALITIES IN THE FETUS AND INFANT

1. One can argue that a condition such as albinism is a metabolic problem visible in the delivery room. It is a problem in the production of skin, hair, and eye pigment. Some malformation syndromes have a metabolic component. They may be diagnosed in the delivery room because of their unusual physical features.

11   ABNORMALITIES IN THE CHILD

1. In children younger than nine, the ratio is normally greater than one. This happens because the head of a normal child is large relative to the rest of the body. The head makes up more of a toddler's height than it does of an adult's height. Standardized charts exist so that comparisons can be made in younger children.

16   TEENAGE ANGST

1. For the record, this author believes that homosexuality, or any other equally complex human behavior, is unlikely to be determined by a single gene. It is much more likely that multiple genes as well as prenatal and postnatal environment each plays a role.

18   GENETICS OF COMMON ADULT DISEASES

1. For example, there is Alzheimer disease (AD) and Lewy body variant of Alzheimer disease (LBV). They both have the same symptoms and involve the same parts of the brain, except that people with LBV have prominent visual hallucinations and certain drug sensitivities that persons with AD do not and there is an extra abnormal feature of the neurons—the presence of Lewy bodies.

Glossary

Abortion Interruption of pregnancy prior to **viability**. This can be spontaneous (also called a miscarriage) or induced.

Acetylcholinesterase (AChE) This is an enzyme that the body makes naturally. It can be measured in amniotic fluid. Increased levels of AChE in amniotic fluid may indicate a problem with the fetus such as a **neural tube defect**.

Achondroplasia The most common form of dwarfism. It is caused by **mutation** in the gene Fibroblast Growth Factor Receptor 3. The gene is on chromosome 4, location 4p16.3. It is an autosomal **dominant genetic disease**. Most cases are caused by new mutations; only a minority are inherited from an affected parent. Achondroplasia has a **paternal age effect**.

Adenine One of the **DNA** bases. Always pairs with **thymine**.

Adult Onset Symptoms of a condition that do not show at all until after a person is an adult.

Advanced Maternal Age Thirty-five years of age. This is the age at which the risk of carrying a fetus with a chromosome problem (1% or 1 chance in 100) is the same as the risk of the amniocentesis procedure.

Advanced Paternal Age About 37 1/2 years. Varies from 35 to 40 years depending upon the reference used. This is more empiric than the definition of **advanced maternal age**.

Allele Plural is "alleles." Alleles are the different forms that a given **gene** can take. All autosomal genes have two alleles. In the population, a given gene may have many different possible alleles, many of which are normal, just different.

Alpha Fetoprotein (AFP) A compound made by the fetus. The specific purpose is unknown, but it may serve as a transport protein in the blood. It crosses the placenta and can be measured in the mother's blood. (AFP is also made by severely diseased livers in adults with cirrhosis or liver cancer.) Increased levels of AFP in the blood of a pregnant woman or in amniotic fluid may indicate a problem with the fetus such as a **neural tube defect**.

Alzheimer Disease A common degenerative brain disease in adults. It usually starts as **dementia** and progresses to a general malfunction of the brain. It is a **multifactorial** disease.

Amino Acid The individual part of a **protein**. The building block of a protein. There are twenty amino acids used in human protein.

Amniocentesis A procedure done on pregnant women to test the **fetus**. A needle is inserted through the woman's abdominal wall and into the uterus. Amniotic fluid is drawn out and can be sent for a variety of tests.

Amyloid Plaque An abnormality in the brain of persons with **Alzheimer disease** and some related conditions. Proteins in the plaque include amyloid and **apolipoprotein E**.

Anencephaly A type of **neural tube defect** in which the skull and brain fail to form correctly. The brain typically degenerates in the uterus. This is a lethal condition.

Aneuploidy Any variation from the normal total number of forty-six chromosomes.

Anticipation Clinical: the recognition that a condition appears earlier or is more severe in subsequent generations. Molecular: worsening of a **repeat mutation** as it is passed from parent to child—the number of repeats increases, further disrupting the gene and its function.

Apolipoprotein E This is a compound found naturally in the body. High levels are associated with heart disease. It is part of the **amyloid plaque** in **Alzheimer disease** There are three forms $e2$, $e3$, and $e4$. The $e4$ form is most associated with Alzheimer disease.

Association A recognized combination of **birth defects** that happen more frequently together than is accounted for by chance alone. A common association is VATER (or VACTERL). The names are acronyms—the letters of the names stand for the birth defects that are part of the association.

Autosomal Dominant A condition inherited in a **dominant** fashion. The gene is on an **autosome**.

Autosome Chromosomes 1 to 22. All the nuclear chromosomes that are not **sex chromosomes**.

Base Pair Two **DNA** bases joined together by weak chemical bonds. One base is on one strand of DNA and the opposing base is on the other strand. The weak chemical bonds between bases hold the two DNA strands together. The bases always pair as A:T and C:G.

Basic Model A way of thinking about **genetic risk** in which everyone has some risk. There are a few people with very low risk, a few people with very high risk, and many people with average risk.

Birth Defect Also called a "congenital anomaly." An abnormality in physical structure that is present at birth. This can be major, such as a missing limb, or minor, such as a skin tag in front of the ear. Can be **genetic** or environmental. Can be **familial**.

Centromere The "waist" of a **chromosome**. It is the point where cellular machinery attaches during **mitosis** and **meiosis**.

Cerebrospinal Fluid The liquid that surrounds and fills the brain and spinal cord. It is constantly circulated and renewed.

Chorionic Villus Sampling A procedure done during **pregnancy** to collect a sample of the placenta.

Chromosome A molecule of **DNA**. Humans have twenty-three pairs of chromosomes twenty-two pairs of **autosomes** and one pair of **sex chromosomes**. Chromosomes are visible under a regular light microscope.

Clinical Geneticist A medical doctor—MD or DO—who has received residency or fellowship training in genetics. In the United States, a medical doctor who is certified by the American Board of Medical Genetics to practice clinical genetics. Someone who provides diagnosis, counseling, and treatment of genetic disease.

Codon Three **DNA** or **RNA** bases in a row in the part of a gene that will undergo **transcription** and **translation**. The codon is the smallest bit of information necessary. Each possible codon specifies a particular **amino acid** in a **protein**.

Cohort A group of individuals who share a particular characteristic, such as age. A classroom of third graders is a cohort.

Compound Heterozygosity The presence of two different **alleles** for one **gene**, both of which are mutated and **pathogenic**. This term is most commonly used in discussions of **recessive** inheritance.

Congenital Present at birth. May be diagnosed by prenatal ultrasound, or may not be discovered until later in life. Can be **genetic** or environmental. Can be **familial**.

Congenital Anomaly *See* **Birth Defect**

Consanguinity/Consanguineous Related by birth. Members of a couple are consanguineous if they have at least one close ancestor in common.

Consultand Person who consults a **clinical geneticist** or **genetic counselor**. This term is most commonly used when the person is a healthy adult, such as a pregnant woman.

Cousin Persons related laterally in a family. First cousins are children of siblings. Second cousins are children of first cousins. Third cousins are children of second cousins, etc. Cousins are "removed" if they are in different generations. Cousins are once removed if there is one generation difference, twice removed if there are two generations difference, etc. (see Figure 2.1).

Cytosine One of the **DNA** bases. Always pairs with **guanine**.

Darwin, Charles (1809–1882) British biologist who observed nature and described the theory of natural selection as the method of evolution. Best known for this work and for his voyages on the H.M.S. *Beagle*.

Deformation A mechanical interference with fetal development that is external to the **fetus** itself. A normally formed fetus is compressed or reshaped by an outside force such as lack of amniotic fluid or uterine fibroids.

Deletion A missing piece of **DNA** at some level. It can be a missing **chromosome**, a piece of a chromosome, or a single missing **base pair**.

Dementia Sign of brain malfunction, including changes in memory, personality, and behavior.

Deoxyribonucleic Acid *See* **DNA**

Developmental Milestone A task or behavior that, when learned, indicates advancing growth and abilities. Common developmental milestones are sitting, speaking words, waving "bye-bye," walking, copying pictures, and sharing.

Diagnostic Testing **DNA** mutation testing or other genetic testing done after symptoms of a disease or condition have manifested.

Disruption An abnormality in fetal development caused by an external chemical, infectious, or radiologic agent. The genetically normal fetus is acted upon by something that disrupts development. **Teratogens** cause disruptions.

Dizygotic Twins Also called "fraternal twins." Two children born from the same **pregnancy** who arise from two different fertilized eggs. Genetically they are only as related as siblings born at different times.

DNA (Deoxyribonucleic Acid) The molecular basis of heredity. A molecule consisting of two phosphate-sugar strands and four different "bases" that project out, joining the two strands together. The bases are **adenine** (A), **thymine** (T), **guanine** (G), and **cytosine** (C). The order of the bases determines the function of a given stretch of DNA. There is also DNA in mitochondria (*see* **Mitochondrial DNA**).

Dominant Genetic Disease Disease that arises in persons **heterozygous**

for a mutation. Only one **allele** of the pair in a gene needs to have a **pathogenic** mutation for the disease to manifest.

Dominant Negative The phenomenon that causes a **dominant genetic disease** when a mutated **allele** actively interferes with the function of the normal allele.

Down Syndrome *See* **Trisomy 21**

Duplication An extra piece of **DNA** at some level. It can be an extra **chromosome**, a piece of a chromosome, or a copied single **base pair**.

Dysplasia An abnormal organization of tissue. Usually confined to one type of tissue, such as bone, cartilage, or kidneys. This is an intrinsic problem in the development of the **embryo** or **fetus**. Dysplasias are often genetic.

Embryo The early-developing organism that arises from some cells of the **zygote**. The embryonic stage is measured from soon after conception through the development of all the major body parts and systems. In humans, the embryonic stage lasts until twelve weeks post conception.

Estriol A naturally occurring compound produced by the placenta and the fetal liver. It can be measured in maternal serum. Low levels of estriol are associated with fetal **trisomy 21**.

Euploid Having the normal number of **chromosomes**.

Evolutionary Conservation Referring to a gene or protein sequence, it is the observation that the sequence is the same in plants and animals of different species. This implies that the sequence is important to the function of the gene or protein. This is particularly true if there are similarities between widely divergent species such as yeasts and mammals.

Expanded Newborn Screening A metabolic test done on a blood sample. In addition to the tests done in routine **newborn screening**, the expanded version tests for fatty acid oxidation disorders such as medium-chain acyl-CoA dehydrogenase (MCAD) deficiency. Expanded newborn screening may test for up to thirty-five different conditions.

Expressivity One way that **dominant genetic disease** can vary from person to person. The difference in disease symptoms from one person to another when they both have the same **mutation** and both show the disease. Compare with **penetrance**.

False Negative A normal test result when disease is really present.

False Positive An abnormal test result when disease is really absent.

Familial Affecting more than one member of the family. Can be **genetic** or environmental. Can be **congenital** or **late onset**.

Fetal Alcohol Syndrome The most common cause of mental retardation.

Estimated to affect up to one in one hundred persons. Caused by maternal intake of alcohol during pregnancy. The full syndrome consists of, at minimum, characteristic facial features, growth retardation, and some functional abnormality of the brain such as mental retardation or seizures.

Fetus The later-developing organism. The fetal stage is measured from the formation of the major body parts and systems until birth. In humans the fetal stage lasts from twelve weeks post conception to thirty-eight weeks post conception.

Folic Acid A B vitamin that functions in **DNA** manufacture and repair. Maternal deficiency in folic acid is associated with the birth defects **spina bifida** and **anencephaly** (**neural tube defects**).

Futility In medicine it is the recognition that a treatment or procedure will not cure a condition. Most often this term is used when a patient is dying and the things that could be done will not really help and may actually increase suffering.

Gamete In higher animals the egg and the sperm are gametes. They are the only cells that normally have half the normal number of **chromosomes**. Gametes from the male and female parent fuse at conception to form the **zygote**.

Gaussian Distribution *See* **Normal Distribution**

Gene A stretch of **DNA** with its promoters and enhancers that, when transcribed in a particular way, leads to the formation of a particular type of **RNA** or a **protein**. A hereditary unit that occupies a specific position within the **genome**; it has one or more specific effects upon the **phenotype** of an organism; it can mutate into various forms, some of which are benign; it can combine with other such hereditary units.

Genetic Caused by a change in the structure of **DNA**. This may be a small change, such as a single base pair **mutation**, or a big change, such as an entire missing or extra **chromosome**. It may be a change in the nuclear (cellular) DNA or in the **mitochondrial DNA**. Not all genetic conditions are **heritable** or **familial**, although most are.

Genetic Code The consecutive **DNA** bases that specify the sequence of **amino acids** in a **protein**. The bases are combined in triplets (**codons**). Each codon specifies a particular **amino acid**.

Genetic Counseling Discussion of **genetic risk** with a patient.

Genetic Counselor A person with a master's degree—MS, MGC, or MSW—who has received specialized training in genetics, specifically in genetic counseling. In the United States, a person who has been certified by the American Board of Medical Genetics or the American Board of Genetic Counselors to practice genetic counseling. Genetic counselors typically work with persons who have already been given a diagnosis or who are at risk for a particular condition.

Genetic Risk The chance that a person, **fetus**, or future **pregnancy** will be affected by a **genetic** condition.

Genetic Sex 46,XX or 46,XY. This may or may not correlate with the **phenotypic sex**.

Genogram A pictorial description of the family history. Used as a tool to diagnose genetic problems and calculate risk. Also called a **pedigree**.

Genome The total complement of genetic material in an individual. This includes both **genes** and noncoding **DNA**.

Genotype The genetic constitution of an individual. In clinical genetics the term is most frequently used to discuss the sequence of a particular **gene**.

Germline Mutation A change in the **DNA** that happens before conception. The change involves the whole body, including the gonads. This type of mutation can be passed on to the next generation.

Gonadal Mosaicism In a **dominant genetic** condition, gonadal mosaicism is the state in which the ovaries of the mother or testes of the father harbor a mutation that is not found anywhere else in the parent's body. Gonadal mosaicism can be a type of **somatic mutation**.

Guanine One of the **DNA** bases. Always pairs with **cytosine**.

Haldane's Method This is a mathematical formula for estimating the relative frequency of **X-linked** mutations in males and females. This is useful for looking at a pedigree and estimating disease recurrence risk. Assuming that the rates of mutation are the same between the sexes, the chance that a new mutation happened in the conception of an affected male is $1/3$. The chance that a new mutation happened in the conception of his mother, who is a carrier, is $2/3$.

Hemizygous The state in a male, or a female with Turner syndrome, in which there are genes on the X **chromosome** when there is no companion **allele** on the Y chromosome. Technically true of the majority of **X-linked** genes, the term is most often used in discussion of **sex-linked diseases**.

Heritable Capable of being passed from parent to child. Usually **genetic**. Can be **congenital** or **late onset**.

Heterozygous The state of having the two **alleles** of a gene be different. One may have a **mutation** while the other is normal. *See also* **compound heterozygosity**.

Homozygous The state of having both **alleles** of a gene be identical. They may both be normal or both have the same **mutation**.

Huntington Disease A neurologic disease affecting mostly adults. It is caused by a mutation in the Huntingtin gene on chromosome 4, location 4p16.3. It is an autosomal **dominant genetic condition**. Essentially all cases are inherited. Huntington disease shows **anticipation** when inherited from one's father.

Hydrocephaly Literally "water brain." An abnormal accumulation of **cerebrospinal fluid** in the skull. Most commonly associated with compression of the brain.

Implantation The attachment of the **embryo** to the uterine inner wall. By definition, the beginning of a **pregnancy**.

Inborn Error of Metabolism A **genetic** condition that causes an abnormality in the way nutrients and other compounds are managed by the body. The vast majority are **recessive genetic diseases**. Common inborn errors of metabolism are phenylketonuria (PKU), galactosemia, and ornithine transcarbamylase (OTC) deficiency.

Informed Consent The process of giving and receiving information. A patient gives consent for a procedure, test, or study after receiving adequate information about the procedure, test, or study, including reasonably predicted risks and benefits. The level of information given is governed by the "reasonable person" standard—what would a reasonable person wish to know prior to a procedure, test, or study.

Intrauterine Growth Restriction Failure of a **fetus** to gain weight and length as expected. Formerly called intrauterine growth retardation.

Inversion A piece of **chromosome** that has been cut out, turned around, and reinserted into place. The term "inversion" can also be used at the **DNA** level. It may be used to describe a turned-around short segment of **base pairs**.

Isolated Birth Defect A structural abnormality of the body, present from birth, that is not accompanied by any other structural defect.

Karyotype A systematized array of **chromosomes** prepared by drawing, photographing, or imaging. A picture that allows analysis of an individual's chromosomes.

Late Onset Conditions manifesting later in life. Can be **genetic** or **environmental**. Can be **heritable**.

Linkage Analysis A method of **genetic** testing or research that determines the presence or absence of a gene **mutation** based upon the surrounding **DNA**. This is used when a gene's location is known but the gene itself has not been characterized or when it is technically difficult to test the mutations directly.

Loss of Function The phenomenon that causes a **dominant genetic disease** when a normal **allele** is insufficient to make up for the **mutation** in and malfunction of the other allele.

Loss of Milestones A child becomes unable to perform a **developmental milestone** that he or she had previously mastered. Loss of milestones is a red flag for **storage disease**.

Lysosome An **organelle** that is essentially a bag of enzymes. The interior of the lysosome is acidic (has a low pH). The lysosome is the place in the cell in which dangerous compounds, bacteria, and other material are broken down.

Malformation An intrinsic problem of embryonic or fetal development. A malformation is a deviation from normal fetal structure. The malformation can be major or minor. Major malformations usually require surgical correction.

Masculinization A condition in females, usually referring to external genitalia that look partially or completely male. For example, a clitoris that is unusually enlarged so that it looks like a penis. Often the result of a **chromosome** or other **genetic** condition.

Maternal Age Effect Influence of maternal age upon the **genotype** or **phenotype** of the offspring. The most commonly recognized maternal age effect is an association between increasing age and increasing risk of chromosomal trisomies—having three copies of a chromosome rather than the normal two.

Maternal Serum Alpha Fetoprotein (MSAFP) Measurement of a compound made by the **fetus** (**alpha fetoprotein**) in a pregnant woman's blood sample. Comparison of the concentration against a normal range can suggest the presence of a problem in the fetus. Too high suggests a **neural tube defect**. Too low can indicate **trisomy 21**.

Medical Ethicist A person who deals with the dilemmas of medicine, such as the conflict between the autonomy of a patient and necessary treatment.

Medical Geneticist A person with a nonmedical doctoral degree—PhD or other—in a human genetics-related field who has received training in medical genetics. In the United States, a person certified by the American Board of Medical Genetics. Medical geneticists may do diagnosis and counseling but will not do treatment.

Medical Specialty An area of medicine in which a doctor receives primary training. Usually the area of residency training.

Medical Subspecialty An area of medicine in which a doctor receives secondary training. Usually the area of fellowship training. Some subspecialties, such as pediatric surgery, are so specific that they are thought of and treated as specialties.

Meiosis The type of cell division that creates the **gametes**—eggs and sperm. The number of **chromosomes** decreases through the phases of meiosis so that the resulting cell (gamete) has half the normal number of chromosomes.

Mendel, Gregor (1822–1884) Moravian monk who worked with garden peas and described the basic patterns of inheritance.

Miscarriage *See* **Abortion**

Mitochondria Singular is "mitochondrion." A subcellular **organelle** primarily responsible for energy production in the cell. It evolved from bacteria and shares characteristics with bacteria. Mitochondria have their own DNA (*see* **Mitochondrial DNA**).

Mitochondrial DNA **Heritable** material found in the **mitochondria**. This **DNA** is circular. One mitochondrion has five to ten copies of DNA in it. All mitochondrial DNA is inherited from the mother in the egg — the sperm does not contribute any mitochondria to the **embryo**.

Mitochondrial Inheritance Also called "maternal inheritance." Describes the way **mitochondria** are passed from one generation to the next. All mitochondria are inherited from one's mother in the egg.

Mitosis Cell division that maintains or increases tissues other than **gametes**. The number of **chromosomes** is maintained from one cell generation to the next.

Monosomy Literally "one body." Having one copy of a chromosome or part of a chromosome instead of the normal two.

Monozygotic Twins Also called "identical twins." Two children arising from the same fertilized egg. They are as closely related genetically as possible in humans, but there will be some differences due to mitochondrial inheritance, postfertilization genetic changes, and developmental differences.

Multifactorial Condition A condition caused by changes in or interaction of many genes and the environment. As opposed to a **single-gene condition**.

Mutation A change in the standard base sequence of **DNA**. Whether this change is good, bad, or neutral depends upon the context.

Organelle A subcellular structure that has a particular function. An organelle is to the cell as an organ is to the body. Some organelles are **mitochondria**, peroxisomes, centrioles, and endoplasmic reticulum.

Neonatal Crash A euphemism to describe a previously healthy newborn who suddenly becomes very sick. Usually happens in the first two or three days after birth. The baby becomes lethargic, stops eating, and has heart and respiratory problems.

Neural Tube Defect (NTD) A birth defect that occurs because the formation of the early brain and spinal cord fails. Neural tube defects are **anencephaly** and **spina bifida**. The risk of neural tube defects can be reduced if a woman takes **folic acid** prior to conceiving a **pregnancy**.

Newborn Screening Also called newborn metabolic screening. Biochemical tests done in the first week of life that look for indications of specific **genetic** diseases. The diseases tested for vary among states in the United States. All states test for phenylketonuria (PKU). Some states use **expanded newborn screening**.

Nondisjunction The failure of **chromosomes** to separate normally during the formation of the **gametes** (**meiosis**). The result is a **trisomy** or a **monosomy**.

Normal Distribution Also called a bell-shaped or **Gaussian distribution**. A commonly used probability model in statistics.

Nucleosome A unit composed of histones with double-stranded DNA wrapped around them. This is the first condensation step of DNA in a cell.

Nucleotide One of the units of **DNA** and **RNA** made up of the bases sugar and phosphate. There are five. In DNA there are deoxyadenylic acid, thymidylic acid, deoxyguanylic acid, and deoxycytidylic acid. In RNA there is uridylic acid instead of thymidylic acid.

Obligate Carrier In **recessive genetic disease**, an obligate carrier is someone who, by default, must have a **mutation**. This person is identified because of the way he or she is related to affected individuals in the family.

Oligogenic A **multifactorial condition** involving just a few genes.

Organelle A structure within the cell that has an identifiable task. Organelles include **mitochondria**, **lysosomes**, peroxisomes, Golgi apparatus, endoplasmic reticulum, etc.

Paternal Age Effect Influence of paternal age upon the **genotype** or **phenotype** of the offspring. The most commonly recognized paternal age effect is an association between increasing age and increasing risk of a new mutation autosomal **dominant genetic disease** such as **achondroplasia**.

Pathogenesis The process of developing a disease, or the way a disease develops.

Pathogenic Disease causing. In genetics this term is used to differentiate a disease-causing **mutation** from a benign **polymorphism**.

Pedigree A formalized family history used in genetics to diagnose and calculate risk for **genetic** disease written out in a standard pictorial form. *See also* **genogram**.

Penetrance In a **dominant genetic disease** it is the likelihood that the disease will manifest if the mutated **gene** is present. Roughly speaking, it is the fraction of people with the **mutation** who show any signs or symptoms of the disease. Compare with **expressivity**.

Percutaneous Umbilical Blood Sampling (PUBS) A procedure performed on a pregnant woman in order to test the **fetus**. A needle is inserted through the woman's abdomen into the uterus and then into the umbilical cord. A sample of fetal blood is obtained and can be sent for various tests. A similar procedure can be used to give the fetus a blood transfusion.

Phenotype The physical characteristics of an individual.

Phenotypic Sex The sex that one appears to be on examination. This may or may not correlate with the **genetic sex**.

Polygenic A **multifactorial condition** involving many genes.

Polymorphism A **mutation** in **DNA** that is present in more than 1% of the population and that is not associated with disease. Different polymorphisms in the same **gene** cause there to be multiple **alleles** for that gene.

Predictive Testing DNA mutation testing done on someone who has a positive family history of disease and who is at risk for the disease but who is not yet showing signs or symptoms.

Pregnancy In a mammalian female, the state that occurs after a fertilized egg (**zygote**) implants into the inner wall of the uterus.

Presymptomatic Someone known or suspected to have a gene **mutation** causing a disease that has not manifested yet.

Primary Relative Someone who shares, on average, 50% (1/2) of their genetic material with the **proband**: parent, child, sibling.

Primary Sexual Characteristics Basic external genital anatomy indicating sex as female or male.

Proband The patient referred for **genetic** diagnosis, counseling, or treatment. Most commonly used to describe a person or **fetus** affected by genetic disease.

Protein A molecule composed of **amino acids** that works in the metabolism or structure of the body.

Recessive Genetic Disease A condition caused by mutation in a **gene** such that both copies of the gene must have a **pathogenic mutation** for the symptoms to manifest.

Reciprocal Translocation An exchange of **genetic** material between two (or more) **chromosomes**. If no net material is gained or lost, this is a balanced **translocation**. If it results in a **duplication** or **deletion** of material, it is unbalanced.

Recombination The swapping of gene **alleles** between sister **chromosomes**. This is a normal process that increases genetic variation from parent to child. There is a small section at each telomere of the X and Y chromosomes that also participates in recombination.

Recurrence Risk Given the presence of a **genetic** condition in a family, recurrence risk is the chance that it will occur in another family member. Recurrence risk varies with inheritance pattern.

Repeat Mutation A change in the **genetic** material that consists of multiple copies of the same two or three **DNA** bases, for example, CGGCGGCGG CGG. A small number is normal. When the repeat expands (grows), it disrupts the function of the **gene**.

Replication Production of a new molecule of **DNA** from an existing one. Production of a new molecule of **RNA** from an existing one (as opposed to **transcription**).

Reverse Transcription The production of a new molecule of **DNA** from an **RNA** template.

Ribonucleic Acid *See* **RNA**

Risk Scientifically, this is different from "chance," which is random. Risk is a statistical estimate that something might or might not happen. It can be calculated if sufficient data are known. The more data that are available for the calculation, the more precise the estimate.

RNA (Ribonucleic Acid) A molecule consisting of one phosphate-sugar strand and four different bases that project out. The bases are **adenine** (A), **uracil** (U), **guanine** (G), and **cytosine** (C). There are three classes of RNA messenger RNA (mRNA), ribosomal RNA (rRNA), and transfer RNA (tRNA). All three classes function in the reading of **DNA** and the production of **proteins**.

Robertsonian Translocation A chromosomal **translocation** in which two **chromosomes** are joined at their **centromeres**. Robertsonian translocations can happen only with chromosomes 13, 14, 15, 21, and 22.

Secondary Relative Someone who shares, on average, 25% (1/4) of their genetic material with the **proband** grandparent, grandchild, aunt, uncle.

Secondary Sexual Characteristics Breast and genital maturation, pubic hair growth, increased stature, alterations in lean body mass, and other changes to the body that take place at puberty.

Sensitivity The ability to identify correctly those who have a disease or a mutation.

Sequence A series of **birth defects** in which the presence of one causes the next. Commonly recognized sequences are holoprosencephaly (primary problem is a brain malformation) and Potter sequence (primary problem is abnormal or absent kidneys).

Sex Chromosomes Chromosomes X and Y.

Sex-Limited Disease A genetic or medical condition that only happens in one or the other sex because the anatomy differs. For example, prostate cancer is a sex-limited disease because it can happen only to males. The genes for these diseases are not necessarily found on the **sex chromosomes**, and they are not necessarily **sex-linked diseases**.

Sex-Linked Disease A genetic condition caused by a mutation of a gene on the X or Y chromosome (the **sex chromosomes**). These conditions are not necessarily limited to one sex or the other—they are not necessarily **sex-limited diseases**.

Sex-Linked Gene A gene found on either of the **sex chromosomes**.

Single-Gene Condition A condition caused by mutation in a specific **gene**. As opposed to a **multifactorial condition**.

Somatic Mutation A change in the **DNA** that takes place in the body after conception. This may cause a **birth defect** or **syndrome**. It may or may not involve the gonads.

Specificity The ability to identify correctly those who do not have a disease or a mutation.

Spina Bifida A **neural tube defect** in which the spine fails to fuse closed. There are two types of spina bifida: meningomyelocele includes a defect in the spinal cord, and meningocele involves just the tissues around the spinal cord. Some cases of spina bifida can be prevented by prenatal use of **folic acid**.

Stillbirth Delivery of a dead fetus or baby after gestational age of **viability**.

Stochastic Randomness or chance.

Storage Disease An **inborn error of metabolism** that results in abnormal accumulation of material in the cell. Accumulation of the material causes the cell to malfunction. Symptoms of the disease depend upon the cells and organs involved.

Syndrome A combination of birth defects that all have the same primary cause.

Technological Imperative The idea that a machine or technology must be used even if it is not the only option. "If we have the machine, we use the machine."

Teratogen A chemical or other agent that causes abnormal development of the **embryo** or **fetus**.

Teratology The branch of science or medicine that studies causes of **birth defects**.

Tertiary Relative Someone who shares, on average, 12.5% (1/8) of their genetic material with the **proband** great grandparent, great grandchild, first cousin.

Threshold Model A way of thinking about genetic risk in which there is no risk of disease until a particular level of liability is reached.

Thymine One of the **DNA** bases. Always pairs with **adenine**.

Transcription The transfer of **genetic** information from **DNA** to **RNA**.

Transducer On an **ultrasound** machine, the hand-held part that creates sound waves and reads how they bounce back.

Translation The creation of a **protein** from the genetic sequence of **RNA**.

Translocation A rearrangement of **genetic** material in large sections. A change in the position of a **chromosome** or part of a chromosome within the **genome**. Translocations can be balanced, having no gain or loss of genetic material, or unbalanced, resulting in a gain or loss of genetic material.

Triplet Three **DNA** bases in a row, such as CGG or AAT. Three bases together may also be called a **codon** if they are in the part of the gene that codes for a protein.

Trisomy Literally "three bodies." Having three copies of any particular chromosome instead of the normal two. *See* **Trisomy 21**

Trisomy 21 A **chromosome** complement in which there are three copies of chromosome 21 rather than the regular two copies. The presence of a third chromosome 21 causes the clinical condition known as Down syndrome.

Ultrasound A medical procedure that employs sound waves to look at physical structure. During **pregnancy** it is used to examine the **fetus**.

Uracil One of the **RNA** bases—used by RNA instead of **thymine**. Always pairs with **adenine** during transcription.

Viability The ability to survive without assistance. For a **fetus** it is usually considered to be 20–24 weeks. The legal definition is often used, which may not correspond to the true viability of the fetus without the mother.

X-Linked A gene physically located on the X chromosome.

Y-Linked A gene physically located on the Y chromosome.

Zygote A fertilized egg. In mammals the zygote divides into multiple cells, some of which become the **embryo** and some of which become the placenta.

Index

Note: Italic page entries refer to tables and figures.

Abortion: induced, 19, 73, 78, 79, 81, 82–84; spontaneous, 19, 43, 44, *44*, 60, 62, 71, 79, 83, 125, 133

Achondroplasia, 13, 54, 68, 104,

Adoption, 81, 84–85

Adrenal hyperplasia, 97, 132, 137

Adult onset genetic disease, 153–154

Advanced maternal age, 74. *See also* Maternal age effect

Advanced paternal age, 68, 71, 74. *See also* Paternal age effect

Alcohol, 12, 13, *22*, 42, 46, *47*, 48, 92, 102, 141

"All or none" period, 42

Allele: Alzheimer disease, 161; autosomal dominant, 52, 53, 54, 56; autosomal recessive, 56, 57, 58, 68; cancer, 163; definition, 35; sex-linked, 63, 124, 125

Alpha fetoprotein (AFP), 76

Alzheimer disease, 159, 160–162, 165

Ambiguous genitalia: female, 131–132; male, 139

American Board of Medical Genetics, 3–4

American College of Medical Genetics, 149

Amino acid, 32–33, 38

Amniocentesis, 77–78, 142

Amniotic band, 90

Amputation, 13, *22*

Amyloid plaque, 160, 161. *See also* Alzheimer disease

Androgen insensitivity syndrome, 133, 134–136, 140

Anencephaly, 82. *See also* Neural tube defect

Aneuploidy, *59*, 142

Anticipation: clinical, 154; molecular, 155

Apert syndrome, 68

Apolipoprotein E, 160–161. *See also* Alzheimer disease

Association, 92–93

Autopsy, 45, 84

Autosomal dominant inheritance. *See* Dominant genetic disease
Autosomal recessive inheritance. *See* Recessive genetic disease
Autosome, 36, 58–62

Bad news, 111–112
Balanced translocation. *See* Translocation
Base pair, *12*, 31
Biotinidase deficiency, 97
Birth defect, *12*, 42, 44, 45, 47, 48, 60, 72, *74*, 75, 76, 81, 84, 89, 90, *91*, 93, 99, 101. *See also* Congenital anomaly
Blood relatives. *See* Consanguinity
Bone age, 104
Breast cancer, 25, 28, 159, 162–164

Capacity, 165–166
Carrier: balanced translocation, 60; recessive mutation, 56–58, 68, 69, 97–99; X-linked mutation, 63, *64*, 71, 72, 122, *122*, 125
Central dogma of biology, 33, *34*
Centromere, 37, 61, *62*, 125
Chorionic villus sampling (CVS), 77, 78–79; and limb defects, 79
Chromosome: abnormality of, 12, 58–62, *59*; 69–71; banding, *37*; condensation, 36; molecules of DNA, *12*, 35, 36; number in humans, 36; structure of, 36–38; testing, prenatal, 78; testing, postnatal, 132
Cleft lip, *17*, 18, 21, *22*, 29, 48, 81, 90, 113, 159
CLIA (Clinical Laboratory Improvement Amendments), 6, 8
Clinical geneticist, 3, 4, 5, 6, 81
Cocaine, 48
Codon, 33
Competent individual, legal definition of, 165, 166, 167

Concussion, 12, *22*, 22, 166
Congenital, definition of term, *12*, 13
Congenital anomaly, *12*, 89. *See also* Birth defect
Connective tissue, 105
Consanguinity, 11, 19, 55, *56*; closed communities, 55
Consequences, 114–115
Consultand, 14. *See also* Proband
Cost of testing, 6–7
Counseling. *See* Genetic counseling
Cousin, 14, *15*, 55, 56, 68
Cystic fibrosis, 25, 69, 105

Death in infancy, 5, *18*, 19, 42, 89
Deformation, 90
Deletion, 59. See *also* Mutation
Dementia, 5, 21, *22*, 160, 161, 167
Deoxyribonucleic acid. *See* DNA
Developmental delay, *18*, 93, 95, 99, 106–109. *See also* Mental retardation
Diagnostic testing, 6
Directive to physicians. *See* Living will
Disruption, 90
DNA (deoxyribonucleic acid) bases, 31, *32*; cancer, 162, 163; as chromosome, 36, 58, 59, 60; function, 32–33; as a gene, 35; history, 31; structure, *12*, 31, *32*, 59–60, 155. *See also* Mitochondrial DNA; Mutation
Dominant genetic disease: and birth defects, 99; definition 51–52; family history of, 52–55; new mutation, 67–68, *74*; pedigree, *52*; recurrence risk, 54, 154; syndromes, 55, 93, 154, 156, 160, 163. *See also* Paternal age effect
Dominant negative mutation, 53
Down syndrome. *See* Trisomy 21

Duplication, 59. See *also* Mutation
Durable power of attorney for health care, 165, 167
Dwarfism, 102, 104
Dysfunction, 89
Dysplasia, 90, 92, 104

Echocardiogram, fetal, 75
Emancipated minor, 146
Environment: condition, 13; in utero, 12, 42, 185; multifactorial disease, 21, 22, *23*, 25–27, 51; teratogen, 45
Estriol, 76
Ethical dilemma, 48, 98, 148, 161
Euploid, *59*
Evolution, 34, 36, 72, 154
Evolutionary conservation, 36
Expanded newborn screening, 96–99
Expressivity, 68, 125. *See also* Penetrance

Failure to thrive, 102, 104–105, *105*
Familial, definition of term, *12*, 13
Familial Alzheimer disease, 160
Familial cancer, 162
Family history, *5*, 13, 14, 18–20, *18*
Fertility, 42–45, 141
Fetal alcohol syndrome (FAS), 12, 13, 42, 92. *See also* Teratogen
Fibrillin, 105
First-degree relatives. *See* Primary relatives
Folic acid: deficiency, 25, 42; Fragile X, 155
45,X, 102, 133–134
47,XXY, 125, 142–143
Fragile X syndrome, 106, 155–156
Futility, 115–116, 168

Galactosemia, 95, 97. *See also* Newborn screening
Gamete, 36, *59*, 60, *61*, *62*, *70*

Gene: definition, 25, 33, 34–35, 152; nomenclature, 25
Genetic code, 33
Genetic counseling, 6, 98
Genetic counselor, 4
Genetic discrimination, concern for, 7
Genetic disease, predominance of, 89
Genetic mystique, 10
Genetic research, 6, 8, 35, 49, 146
Genetic risk, prediction of, 18, 19, 25. *See also* Dominant genetic disease; Recessive genetic disease; Sex-limited disease; Sex-linked disease
Genetic sex, 126, 132, 134, *135*, 141
Genetic testing, 6; by ethnic group, 69; Huntington disease, 156–157; of minors, 148–149
Genetics: cause of pregnancy loss, 62; definition, *12*; in prenatal testing, 74, 78, 79. *See also* Dominant genetic disease; Recessive genetic disease; Sex-limited disease; Sex-linked disease
Genogram. *See* Pedigree
Genome, 25, 34, 35, 169
Genotype, 134, 157
Germ theory of disease, 21
German measles. *See* Rubella
Glycogen storage disease, 108
Gonadal mosaicism, 68
Growth hormone, 102, 104, 109, 134

Haldane's method, 71
Hearing screening, 107–108
Heart disease, 21, 26–27, *27*, 161
Hemihyperplasia, 106
Hemizygous/Hemizygosity, 63, 123, 124, 125, 134

Hemophilia, 11, 71, 79
Heritable/Heritablility, 11, *12*, 13, 67
Heterozygous/Heterozygosity, 35, 53, 54, 57, 58
Histones, 36
Homocystinuria, 106
Homosexuality, 147
Homozygous/Homozygosity, 35, 54, 57, 58, 125
Hospice, 116–117, *117*
Human chorionic gonadotropin (hCG), 76, 141
Human Genome Project, 34, 35
Huntington disease, 13, 153–157. *See also* Triplet repeat
Hypospadias, 139–141
Hypothyroidism, 97

Implantation, 42
Incompetent individual, legal definition of, 165, 166
Infertility, 5, *22*, 93 140; in Androgen insensitivity syndrome, 136; in Klinefelter syndrome, 142, 143; pregnancy loss, 41, 154; in Turner syndrome, 132, 134
Informed assent, 145, 146
Informed consent 8, *9*, 77
Internet medical information, 7
Inversion, *59*
Isolated birth defect, 67, 90, 93
IVF (in vitro fertilization), 18

Karyotype, 38
Klinefelter syndrome. *See* 47,XXY
Knudson hypothesis, 163

Language: delay in, 107; developmental milestone, 107; hearing problems and, 107, 108
Late onset disease, *12*, 13
Legal guardian, 165, 166–167
Linkage analysis, 156
Living will, 165, 167–168

Lottery, 23, *24*
Lyon, Mary, 125
Lyonization, 125
Lysosomal storage disease, 108
Lysosome, 108

Magical thinking, 113
Male-to-male inheritance, *52*, 63, *64*, 122
Malformation, 89, 90, 93, 101, 133
Manifesting carrier, 122, 125
Maple syrup urine disease, 95, 97
March of Dimes, 7, 97
Marfan syndrome, 105–106
Marriage 11, 19, 55
Masculinization of female, 131
Mass spectrometry. *See* Expanded newborn screening
Maternal age effect, 70. *See also* Advanced maternal age
Maternal inheritance, 65. *See also* Mitochondria
Maternal serum alpha fetoprotein (MSAFP), 76
Maternal serum screen, 73, 76–77
MCAD (medium-chain acyl-coenzyme A dehydrogenase), 97
Measurements, 5
Medical ethicist, 116
Medical specialty, 3, 4, 5
Medical subspecialty, 3
Meiosis, 60, *70*
Mendel, Gregor, 34, 38
Mendelian inheritance, 34, 38
Mental retardation, *18*, 22, *22*, 106, 134, 166. *See also* Developmental delay
Metabolic disease, 93–95
Mifepristone, 83
Milestones: developmental, 106–107; loss of, 108
Miscarriage. *See* Abortion, spontaneous
Mitochondria, 63, 65

Mitochondrial DNA (mtDNA), 63, 66
Mitochondrial inheritance, 63–66, 65, 99
Mitosis, 36
Model, construction of, 28
Monosomy X. *See* 45,X
MSAFP. *See* Maternal serum alpha fetoprotein
Müllerian inhibiting factor, 136
Multifactorial condition: adult onset disease, 159, 160; cancer, 162; definition, 22, 25–27, *26, 27*; and environmental factors, *23*; recurrence risk, 28–29; types of birth defects, 93
Mutation: cancer, 162–164; carrier of, 122; definition, *12*, 53, 67; dominant, 52, 54, 67, 68; gain of function, 53; loss of function, 53; mitochondrial DNA, 63, 65; recessive, 25, 56–58, 68–69; repeat, 153, 155, X-linked, 63, *64*, 71, 72, 122, 123, 124, 125

Neonatal crash, 94
Neural tube defect, 77, 92
Neurofibromatosis, 54
Newborn screening, 95, *96*, 98, 106, 132. *See also* Expanded newborn screening
Nondisjunction, 69, 70, *70*, 71, 142. *See also* Maternal age effect
Nucleosome, 36

Obligate carrier, 122, *122*
Oligogenic, 22
Organelles, 63, 96, 108
Osteogenesis imperfecta, 104
Overgrowth, 106

p arm, 37
Paternal age effect, 68, 71, *74*. *See also* Advanced paternal age
Pathogenesis, 89, 159

Peas, 34
Pedigree: cancer, 163; construction of, 15–18; dominant, *52*; recessive, *56*; relatedness, 14; X-linked, *64*, 122, *122*
Penetrance, 122, 125. *See also* Expressivity
Percutaneous umbilical blood sampling (PUBS), 79
Phenotype, 35
Phenotypic sex, 134
Photographs, taking of, 5, 146
Pierre Robin sequence, 92
PKU (phenylketonuria), *49*, 95, 97. *See also* Newborn screening
Poland anomaly, 133
Polycystic kidney disease, 54, *55*
Polygenic conditions, 22
Potter sequence, 92
Prader-Willi syndrome, 106, 140
Predictive testing, 156, 157
Pregnancy: dating of, 42, *43*; definition of, 42; likelihood of, 44; loss of, 19, 41, 43, 45; tests for, 43; timing of, 45. *See also* Implantation; Unplanned pregnancy
Premutation, 155, 156. *See also* Triplet repeat
Prenatal screening, 73
Prenatal testing, *74*
Presymptomatic, 148. *See also* Predictive testing
Primary relatives, 14, *14*, 160
Primary sexual characteristics: female, 126, 131, 133; male, 126, 142
Proband, 13. *See also* Consultand
Protein, 32–33, *34*
Proteome Project, 35
PUBS. *See* Percutaneous umbilical blood sampling

q arm, 37

Recessive genetic disease: and birth
defects, 99; cancer, 163;
definition of, 56, 57; and ethnic
group, 69; family history of, 55;
metabolic disease, 97, 108; new
mutation, 56; pedigree, 56;
recurrence risk, 57, 57, 58
Reciprocal translocation, 60, 61
Recombination, 36, 37, 126, 155
Recurrence risk: dominant, 54, 68;
mitochondrial, 65; multifactorial,
28, 29; prediction of, 66;
recessive, 57, 69; X-linked, 64;
Y-linked, 64
Referral for genetic services, 5
Relatedness, 14, 15
Removed, cousins, 14, 15
Repeat mutation, 153, 155–156.
See also Triplet repeat
Replication, 33
Research labs, 6, 8
Research studies, participation in,
7–10
Retrovirus, 33
Reverse transcription, 33
Ribonucleic acid. See RNA.
Right not to know, 148–149
Risk: Basic Model, 26, 27;
prediction of, 18, 23–25, 28–29;
Threshold Model, 26, 28
RNA (ribonucleic acid), 33, 34
Robertsonian translocation, 60, 61,
62
Roe v. Wade, 84
RU-486. See Mifepristone
Rubella, 47, 47

Saunders, Cicely, 116
Schizophrenia, 22, 68, 160
Screening, 69, 76, 97. See also
Hearing screening; Newborn
screening; Prenatal screening
Second-degree relatives. See
Secondary relatives

Secondary relatives, 14, 14
Secondary sexual characteristics:
female, 126, 131, 134; male,
126, 142
Sensitivity, 6
Sequence, 90, 92
Sex chromosomes, 36, 63, 121–125,
126, 133–135, 142–143
Sex-limited disease, 121
Sex-linked disease, 63, 64, 71,
121–126
Sex-linked gene, 63, 64
Short stature: disproportionate,
102, 104; proportionate, 102
Sickle cell, 69, 95, 97
SIDS (sudden infant death
syndrome), 48, 97
Skeletal dysplasia. See Short stature,
disproportionate
Skipping a generation, 51
Smoking, 22, 25, 28, 42, 48, 162
Social Darwinism, 12
Somatic mutation, 67, 125
Specificity, 6
Spina bifida, 21, 28, 42, 76,
66, 78, 81, 82, 92, 108, 113.
See also Neural tube defect
Statistical risk, 23–25
Stillbirth, 5, 18, 19, 44, 60
Stochastic factors, 25, 25, 26, 26
Storage disease, 108
Surrogate decision maker, 166, 167
Susceptibility, 13, 162, 163
Syndrome, 5, 13, 68, 91–92, 93,
102

Tall stature, 105–106
Tandem mass spectrometry. See
Expanded newborn screening
Tanner, J. M., 126
Tanner stages, 126–128; female,
127, 128; male, 128, 128
Tay-Sachs disease, 69
Technological imperative, 115

Teratogen, 45–48, *47*, 83, 90, 102
Teratogenicity, 45, 46
Teratology, 45
Tertiary relatives, 14, *14*
Testicular feminization. *See*
  Androgen insensitivity syndrome
Testis determining factor (TDF),
  126, 135
Thalidomide, 46
Third-degree relatives. *See* Tertiary
  relatives
Transcribe/Transcription, 33, 36,
  125
Translate/Translation, 33, 36
Translocation: balanced, 59, 60
  chromosome, 59, 69; reciprocal,
  60, *61*; Robertsonian, 61, *62*;
  unbalanced, 60, 62
Triplet repeat, 155–156. *See also*
  Codon; Premutation
Triploidy, *59*
Trisomy 13, 71
Trisomy 16, 62
Trisomy 18, 71
Trisomy 21: adoption, 84;
  chromosome problem, 13, 38,
  61, 69, *70*, 71, 92; Down

syndrome, 92, 93, 112, 140,
  160, 167; frequency of, 59;
  prenatal testing for, 76, 77;
  recurrence, 12, 142
Turner syndrome, 62, *70*, 102, 125,
  133–134. *See also* 45,X

Ultrasound, 6, 41, 82, 132; prenatal
  testing and, 73, 75, 77, 78 79
Unplanned pregnancy, 41, 42
Uracil. *See* RNA

Vaccinations, 46
VATER association, 92
Viability, 83

X inactivation, 125
X-linked diseases, *52*, 63, *64*, 71,
  121–126, *122*, *123*, *124*;
  androgen insensitivity syndrome,
  134–135, *135*; Fragile X
  syndrome, 155
XIST gene, 125

Y-linked diseases, 63, *64*, *126*

Zygote, 42, 43, 44, 60, 65, 69

About the Author

ANGELA SCHEUERLE, M.D., is a Clinical Geneticist in private practice, as well as Medical Director for the Texas Birth Defects Research Center. She is also Medical Director for the Dallas Craniofacial Center and Genetics Medical Center. She is a Faculty Member for the Program of Ethics in Science and Medicine at the University of Texas Southwestern Medical School. Scheuerle is also an Adjunct Faculty Member at the School of Public Health at the University of Texas and a Volunteer Faculty Member for the Clinical Ethics in Medicine course at the University of Texas Southwestern Medical School at Dallas.